"Thank you, Elle, for writing this joyous, funny and very educational guide to doing it and doing it right. *Curvy Girl Sex* had me laughing out loud dreaming about executing positions I'd never heard of. I loved this book and feel like it was written just for me. You will, too. Now let's get to bangin'!"

—**Bridget Everett**, singer, actor, writer, comedian

"*Curvy Girl Sex* is a must-read! From positions and dirty talk to solo-sex and body image, Elle offers practical advice you can use tonight—in and out of the bedroom. This will be my new go-to guide for sexual positions for every body."

—**Jessica O'Reilly**, Ph.D., best-selling sex author, www.SexWithDrJess.com

"Elle Chase sizzles with big, beautiful, brave energy as a sex educator and author. *Curvy Girl Sex* is filled with creative positions parallel to the Kama Sutra."

—**Dr. Ava Cadell**, author of *Idiot's Guides: Kama Sutra* and founder of Loveology University

"Elle Chase is her own best advertisement. Funny, wise, kind, and compassionate, she is an excellent counselor and coach. She's walked the walk and now she wants to share what she's learned with clients who are ready to be happy, whole, and healthy. Highly recommended!"

—**Nina Hartley**, author of *Nina Hartley's Guide to Total Sex*

"Elle Chase has risen up to become one of the most proficient sex educators today. Online, she has helped pioneer conversation around smut, body image, and sex after 40. You won't find a more honest and authentic educator, one who can speak from the heart and the brain."

—**Jamye Waxman**, author of *Getting Off: A Woman's Guide to Masturbation*

"Elle is a remarkable blend of warm openheartedness and sexy braininess. Provocative and judgment free, she creates a safe space for people to explore their own minds and bodies without shame and with a lot of love, knowledge, and compassion. She is a true gift to the sex-positive sex-education world."

—**Melissa White**, CEO, www.LuckyBloke.com

"Elle Chase writes and teaches about sex as fun and humorous as it is. She is knowledgeable, enthusiastic, and passionate about teaching sexuality."

—**Tara Struyk**, editor, www.kinkly.com

"Elle Chase is an incredibly dedicated and gifted presenter, writer, and educator. Believing that everyone is entitled to a safe, hot, healthy sex life, she has made it her life's work to provide workshops and lectures where sex positive adults can exchange ideas openly, free of judgment."

—**Jaeleen Bennis**, creator and founder of Bondassage

"I can think of no other sex positive educator I want to simultaneously seek advice from and share a cup of coffee with than Elle Chase. She is often SheVibe.com's go-to expert for brainy sex advice and articles; she never fails to deliver."

—**Sandra Bruce**, partner, www.SheVibe.com

"With candor, wit, and gentleness, Elle Chase begins with the assumption that sexuality is not exclusive to cover models— which is great, because very few of us are. Then, pairing data with real warmth, Chase helps readers and clients find comfort in their own skin."

—**Gram Ponante**, journalist, author, and writer, www.GramPonante.com

"Elle Chase is our go-to expert for articles about sex topics that really matter to our readers. Her deep knowledge base combined with a no-nonsense, humorous style make her approachable and completely reliable."

—**Paula Tiberius**, editor, www.sexpert.com

"Elle Chase approaches sex from all directions with candor, vulnerability, and above all else, a fantastic smile on her face. Her work is a pleasure and an education all in one experience."

—**Jon Pressick**, www.SexInWords.ca

Curvy Girl

SEX

101 BODY-POSITIVE POSITIONS
TO EMPOWER YOUR SEX LIFE

Elle Chase

FAIR WINDS

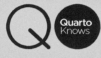

Inspiring | Educating | Creating | Entertaining

Brimming with creative inspiration, how-to projects, and useful information to enrich your everyday life, Quarto Knows is a favorite destination for those pursuing their interests and passions. Visit our site and dig deeper with our books into your area of interest: Quarto Creates, Quarto Cooks, Quarto Homes, Quarto Lives, Quarto Drives, Quarto Explores, Quarto Gifts, or Quarto Kids.

First Published in 2015 by Fair Winds Press, an imprint of The Quarto Group, 100 Cummings Center, Suite 265-D, Beverly, MA 01915, USA. T (978) 282-9590 F (978) 283-2742 QuartoKnows.com

Fair Wind Press titles are also available at discount for retail, wholesale, promotional, and bulk purchase. For details, contact the Special Sales Manager by email at specialsales@quarto.com or by mail at The Quarto Group, Attn: Special Sales Manager, 100 Cummings Center, Suite 265-D, Beverly, MA 01915, USA.

ISBN: 978-1-59233-740-8

Library of Congress Cataloging-in-Publication Data available

Cover and book design: Laia Albaladejo

Photography: Nick Holmes

Endpaper credits: Erin Nelson, Alexis Cathleen and Rae of Sunshine Photography, Amy Hunter, Zane, Dawn Serra, Emma Dowell, Jennifer Barreto-Leyva, Isobel Roberts, Kenna Lee, K.L. Joy and Darren Clarke, Luna Matatas, Mistress Kay, Rebecca Hiles, Renée Romano, and Red Hot Suz

Illustrations: Jenn St-Onge and Kimmy Hutchison

Model: April Flores

Hair and Make Up: Victor Del Castillo

To Tristan, JoEllen, Anne, Cyndi, Jemma, Shannon, and Justin for all their unending support, smarts, and love.

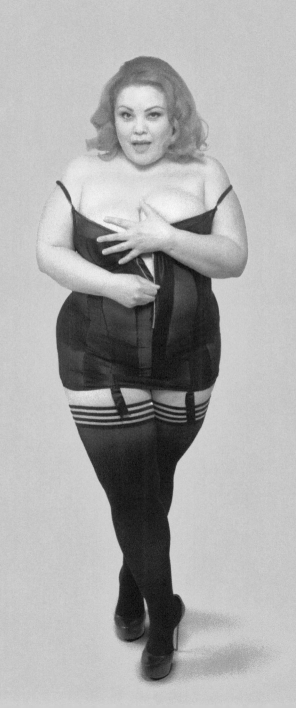

Contents

Preface

I became a sex educator and body acceptance advocate by accident. Fresh out of a seven-year marriage where there was barely any sex, I craved passion—which I saw on TV and movies, but never experienced in my own life. Never feeling desirable, sexy, or worthy of sexual pleasure, I had always felt neuter, unconnected to my body and convinced that sex and the joys that came with a good sex life were for other people, not me.

I was desperate for passion. So after I left my husband, I had a conundrum. I was single, overweight, and completely unequipped with the tools to date successfully or to have passionate, confident sex without caring about how fat I was. I longed to feel someone crave me. But, I thought, who could feel passion for a fat chick, with cellulite, scars, florescent-white skin, and crooked teeth? I had always believed that people like me didn't experience high-adrenaline, fervent, ardent love affairs. In the past, I felt I had to be realistic, had to accept that I would never be the object of the desire and salacious abandon that I craved. I assumed I had to settle for what I could find and somehow make it work.

But I was wrong. Oh boy, was I wrong.

Because my desire for passion was overwhelming, I felt I had nothing to lose, so I started dating online. Sure, I got rejected just like everyone does, but what I discovered was that all types of men were interested in me. Some of them had a penchant for my body type, some men didn't care about body type, and some men found the whole package attractive. This was a revolutionary concept to me. I didn't expect to sleep with or date such a variety of fascinating, smart, and passionate men—of all shapes and sizes. I went out with "traditionally good-looking" actors, a super-sexy masseur, a politician, a nerdy techie, and a dashing photographer, to name a few. Most of these men were younger than me, and not only were all of them physically and personally different, they were also all attracted to me regardless of my weight and "flaws." My belief that I was inherently undesirable quickly evaporated.

I realized that not only was I attracted to all types of men—tall, short, fat, skinny, long-haired, bald, scarred, smooth, muscled, soft—but that these men were attracted to me. If this was true in *my* life, I couldn't be the only one. This realization gave me the germ of self-confidence that I needed to further explore and experience the sexual passion I so desired and, in a short time, got. I realized my judgment that I was unattractive and undesirable wasn't based in reality; it was a verdict I came to subconsciously over a lifetime of feedback and opinions gathered from mean girls at school, the media, and some really poor choices in men. The truth was, I was sexy as hell. As long as I didn't pay attention to my old misconceptions, and instead focused on enjoying myself, which included discovering what (and who) made me feel sensual and sexy, how to identify it in my body, the ways I feel chemistry with someone, and how to recognize when they were feeling it, too.

During this time, I came to understand that the negative feelings I had toward my body and my sexual desirability was a social construct thrust upon me—one that I unwittingly and subconsciously took part in. I finally understood that this construct—that fat women aren't sexy, or a woman must wear heels and flirty dresses, that she must bat her eyes and let her date determine her dateability—was a lie. I was *free*. I wanted all women to know this fact. I wanted all women to know—and feel confident—that we are *all* sexy, and it has nothing to do with flat abs or lustrous hair, but everything to do with how sexy we *feel* and how connected we are to our sexuality.

This truth was the impetus for this book. You can't enjoy sex if you're constantly worrying about whether you're sexy enough for your partner. You can't enjoy sex when you are thinking about how to do it while looking elegant or hiding your rolls. You can't enjoy sex if your mind is wandering and you're not concentrating on your partner's pleasure and your own. This is more than a book of sex positions. I hope that this book will show you how to own and accept your body the way it is right now . . . and then move on and have a fulfilling sex life.

I hope that in some way this book will empower you to not let anything get in the way of improving your sex life. Whether you learn a new position or two, come away with a better understanding of your pleasure or anatomy, or go out and buy your first sex toy, it'll be a great step to a richer sex life. Regardless, know that you deserve pleasure and it's never too late to find it!

Introduction

Accepting your body means accepting that sexual pleasure is not just meant for other people. Sex is a human right. Take back that right! Empower yourself as a sexy, sensual woman by discovering your likes and dislikes, turn-ons and turn-offs, and the positions that give you the most pleasure. This book is chock full of great positions, whether you're a beginner who is just starting to venture away from missionary position, or an advanced sexual partner who is looking for even more ways to experiment. There are also fun facts throughout the book, including sexual health information, advice on which toys will make your sex life sing, communication tips, and much more. Let's take a tour, shall we?

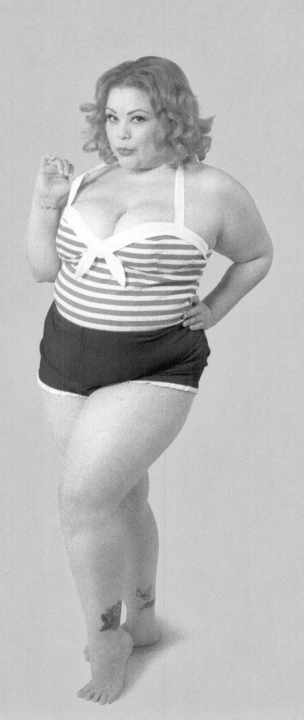

About the Positions in this Book

All positions were chosen because they either tend to be easier for women of size to get into, or the positions open up the genital area of the receiver, making access to the vulva/vagina/anus much easier. Sometimes greater access is useful, but you might need some extra assistance to make a position more comfortable. For many positions you'll find "Elle's Big Move," which explains how to adapt positions to make them more pleasurable or take them to the next level. These as well as Chapter 2, Sex Toys and Other Sexy Essentials, offer some solutions to whatever comfort and ability concerns you might have. But at the end of the day, you're still going to have to move any flesh and folds that make a particular position challenging. Yes, I just said "flesh" and "folds."

Not every position will work for you. In fact, if this book gives you just a few new positions you enjoy, I'd call that a success. After all, changing up your routine with a partner can be challenging. You might find new positions that are simply too demanding right now, but don't fret. Barring any health limitations, you can perform stretches and become more flexible to eventually perform more advanced poses. The fact of the matter is that the positions you might see porn stars doing are not positions the rest of us can do right off the bat, if at all. Porn actors are professionals—in fact, think of them as trained athletes. You wouldn't expect to wake up on a Sunday morning and run a marathon without any training, would you? Athletic accomplishments, including sexual ones, take skill and practice.

Try and think about tackling new positions like learning new dance moves. At first it feels awkward and you may make missteps or feel clumsy, but once you get the hang of it, you can incorporate these new moves like they've always been part of your repertoire. Though 101 positions is a lot, it's not an exhaustive list. You may find yourself trying a position in the book and then coming up with your own modifications or hacks, and to that I say, "Good for you! Spread the word! Tell your friends!"

The Versatility of Pillows

You're going to hear me endlessly sing the praises of pillows for a majority of the positions in this book, for good reason. They make sex easier in so many ways. If you have a big butt and you're the bottom partner, placing a pillow under your hips will take the pressure off your lower lumbar. If you're trying downward doggy style and your boobs are feeling squished, try placing a pillow under them. Using supports under your bum or under your tum to raise your hips to meet your lover's cock or strap-on provides greater access for entry and enables gravity to help fleshy parts pull away from the genitals as well.

When using pillows, make certain that they are firm enough to elevate the hips at least 6 inches (15 cm); you can go lower or higher depending on comfort. A pillow (or a couple of them) can tilt your hips high enough to let gravity direct flesh away from the genitals.

A lot of people use bed pillows, but bed pillows don't usually offer enough support because they are easily flattened, especially after a long bout of lovemaking. Sofa cushions or throw pillows are better choices for getting down, as they are probably the firmest pillows you'll have available. Personally, I find that the industrial foam used in the Liberator sex furniture products, particularly the Wedge and Ramp, support me more reliably. The Wedge is small enough to store under the bed, and the Ramp can be popped in a closet for easy (and discreet) access. See the Curvy Resources section on page 178 for more information on Liberator. No matter what you decide to use—a Liberator or a pillow—supports are truly a curvy girl's best friend.

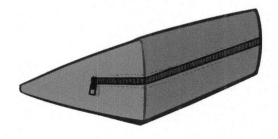

Giver, Receiver, Pronouns, and Bodies

When discussing the partners in a position, I will use words that describe functional anatomy—not gender. I've made the choice to refer to the partner doing the penetrating as "the giver" and the partner being penetrated as "the receiver" instead of "man" and "woman." Here's why:

1. Not everyone with a vulva and vagina identifies as female, and not everyone with a penis identifies as male.
2. You don't need to have a penis to penetrate your partner. Strap-on harnesses with dildos can be used by either partner to enter a vagina or anus.
3. In the same vein, you don't need a vagina to be penetrated. Everyone has a butt, and people of all gender expressions enjoy putting things in them. (More about that later.)
4. There are some people who don't identify as a male or a female at all. They may identify as agender, genderqueer, gender fluid, or nonbinary.

Gender pronouns, such as she/he and her/him, will be used interchangeably throughout the book.

Please note that just because a partner is referred to as "he" does not mean it is required or assumed that the partner must be male. Similarly, a variety of genders and couples will be illustrated to show how each position is performed. If your gender or coupling differs from what is illustrated or described, but you have the anatomy or toys to make it work, go for it!

I sometimes use the word "fat," as I consider it to be an accurate descriptor of some curvy gals, including myself. I believe using "fat" in a nonpejorative way helps destigmatize and inure us to the word as the insult it's become, and gets us used to seeing it as it was meant to be used: as a neutral descriptor. I use the words curvy, plus-size, zaftig, rounder, plump, larger, and bigger in the same spirit. Some of these words may make you bristle at first, but they are not meant negatively, just as adjectives.

We assume that if you're reading this book, you identify as, or have a partner who identifies as, a curvy girl—regardless of gender or anatomy. Rest assured that you'll find plenty of positions that will work for you or that can be adapted accordingly.

Pregnant Women

I've included pregnant women in this book because a lot of these positions are useful when the expectant mom's tummy becomes a challenge while having sex. However, the difference between a big pregnant stomach and having a big stomach is important. A pregnant tummy pretty much stays in one place and doesn't have any give like a fleshy tummy does, so it can't be manipulated in the same ways. Also, there's a living thing in there, so there are different precautions to worry about. If you're pregnant, remember that *you* are the authority on your own body. Only do what is comfortable and pleasurable, and what your health care provider says is acceptable for you and the health of your pregnancy.

Trans Men and Women

We live in a world where some curvy girls may be transitioning or may have already transitioned into the voluptuous women they are. GLAAD, the Gay and Lesbian Alliance Against Defamation, defines "transgender" as "a term used to describe people whose gender identity differs from the sex the doctor marked on their birth certificate. Gender identity is a person's internal, personal sense of being a man or a woman (or someone outside of that gender binary). For transgender people, the sex they were assigned at birth and their own internal gender identity do not match."

Trans women come in all shapes and sizes and with varying genitalia and may have opted to keep their penis intact; thus I have written this book to include trans women as well.

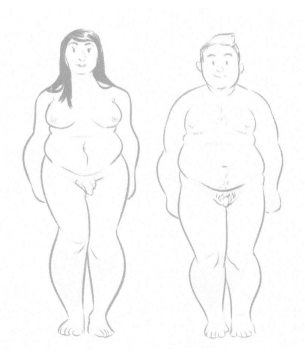

About This Book

You might notice that the positions don't start until the middle of this book. What gives? This book is not just about getting into comfortable positions. After all, there is much more to enjoy, explore, and learn about curvy-girl sex than where to put your bodies and parts. Some chapters that might not seem immediately self-explanatory are some of my favorites.

The first chapter, Every Body is Built for Pleasure, talks about how sexiness has been defined throughout the ages and about discovering how *you* define it out in the world and in yourself. It also briefly covers some pleasure anatomy, how it works, and why arousal and foreplay are so important to good sex. Chapter 2, Sex Toys and Other Sexy Essentials, covers just that: fun things to use while you're having fun.

Chapter 3, Curvy Girl Prep: Sensuality, Communication, and Getting in the Mood, is all about getting in the mood—mentally, physically, and sensually—for a night of passion. It includes methods for tuning into your five senses to get your juices flowing, as well as some erotica and porn recommendations. In this chapter, you will learn how to discover your unique sensuality and how to use it to build confidence—and thus, enhance intimacy with your partner.

And finally (you waited so patiently), you'll find several chapters of positions—from those you may already be familiar with (plus some fun variations) and solo sex techniques, to oral sex positions and other ways to get it on. You'll find 101 positions in total to help you broaden your sexual horizons.

Finally, there is a comprehensive Curvy Resources section, directing you to the products listed in this book as well as other sexually relevant materials, sites, books, companies, organizations, and professionals that a curvy girl might need.

Organizational Icons

Because a lot of us curvy gals have different areas on our bodies that can challenge us during sex, I've come up with a key of handy-dandy, color-coded icons to let you know what positions might be best for you. Does the junk in your trunk concern you? Just look for the green tushy icon under the position name for tush-friendly positions. Does your back ache when you're trying to get down? Just find the navy-blue back icon and you're good to go! I've also included icons that indicate what positions might be good for anal sex, pregnancy, or to use with a harness. So have a gander below and make note of the icon or icons that you feel apply to you.

 Easier on the back

 Easier on the knees

 Easier on the arms

 Easier on the giver

 Easier on the receiver

 If you have a big partner

 Good position for anal sex

 Suitable for pregnant women

 Strap-on friendly

 Easier for women with a larger stomach

 Easier for women with larger thighs

 Easier for women with a larger butt

What I Wish Someone Had Told Me about Sex as a Fat Chick

1. You are inherently sexy. You were born with it. Just like the color of your hair or the shape of your fingers, your sexiness comes factory installed. You can cover it up, ignore it, or try to deny its existence, but it doesn't go away.

2. A person is sexy because they know and believe they are. How do you build sexual self-confidence? The same way you get to Carnegie Hall: practice, practice, practice. Start incrementally if you need to—just start.

3. There's a pot for every cover. If people were only attracted to a standard set of qualities and characteristics, the human race would have died out eons ago. Our diversity—what makes us different—is what most people respond to.

4. Your partner knows what you look like and wants to be there. One-night stand or long-term lover—if your partner didn't think you were sexually attractive, chances are they wouldn't be having sex with you. End of story.

5. Some things you just have to be okay with or decide not to think about in bed—number one is how you look. Your body shape, weight, and extra pounds are inconsequential when it comes to doing the deed. Fat, bodies, positions, and mobility can all be manipulated in order to get down. Don't waste precious sexy time worrying about it. It distracts from your own pleasure and that of your partner. Try your best to be in the moment.

6. You need to have sex to feel better about your body during sex, and this includes solo sex. As long as you get those juices flowing on a regular basis by someone else's hand, or your own, you're exercising your sexual self. The more you get used to being in a sexual state in your body, the faster you'll get used to it.

7. Sex can be inelegant under the best circumstances. But, if you communicate honestly with your partner in the beginning, you're setting the stage for your sexual relationship to keep growing. High fives for everyone!

Get Started

I can't reiterate enough that the courage, confidence, and ability needed to hold up your belly, manipulate your thighs with your hands, pull your butt cheeks apart, or readjust your boobs is essential. Hopefully, the organizational icons and the chapters that precede the positions sections will help you get there if you're not already. By the end of this book, I hope you'll feel more confident about your curvy body and totally empowered to have hot, steamy sex in a variety of ways!

Chapter

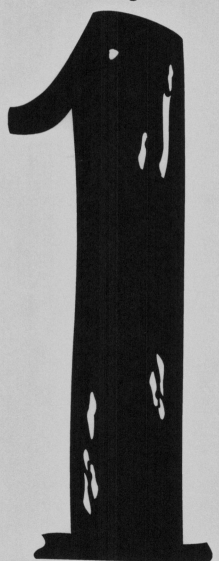

Adequate arousal is essential for two reasons. One is that it prevents injury, which can totally be avoided with proper preparation. The second—and potentially more helpful reason—is that allowing time and headspace for satisfactory arousal means everything feels so much better. Full arousal can be the difference between "Meh" sex and "My goodness, that was fucking outstanding."

Cyndi Darnell, sex and relationship therapist

Every Body is Built for PLEASURE

The History of Sexy Curvy Gals

Throughout history women's bodies have been painted, sculpted, and drawn in a variety of different sizes, shapes, and characteristics—evidence of a wide definition for what was considered appealing at any particular time. Larger women in particular have been deemed the height of sexual desirability at many points in history: from the plump and fleshy women Peter Paul Rubens represented in his Baroque paintings, to the exaggerated large men and women Fernando Botero depicted in the 1950s, to the voluptuous hourglass bombshells motion pictures made famous in the 1960s. For several decades, a thinner physique was the apex of sexual desirability, but today, curvy is back! More curvy women are accepting, even loving, their bodies as they are, flaunting their luscious curves, their ample tummies, and their bodacious butts and breasts. Together, we're rallying companies to carry more sizes of chic and stylish clothes, and fashion houses are responding not only by extending their size ranges in existing ready-to-wear collections but by also creating clothing lines with curvy women in mind.

Entertainment and media conglomerates are finally recognizing that curvy women are desirable, viable, bankable and sought-after sexual beings. Melissa McCarthy is carrying her own movies with top billing, and plus-size models have graced the covers of top fitness and fashion magazines, including Ashley Graham on the cover of the famed *Sports Illustrated* swimsuit issue. As a community, we have expanded everyone's idea of what a sensual, sexy, sexual, beautiful, smart, empowered, modern woman looks like. *We* are showing the world how sexy we are, and boy, is it listening.

What Is Sexy?

Good question. I'm glad you asked. YOU! *You* are sexy! Everyone is sexy. I believe that "sexy" is an attribute, something we are all born with. You may have heard it a million times, but sexiness is how we project what and how we feel. Now, this next part is important.

We *all* have sex appeal, but our sex appeal is not going to be everyone's definition of sexy. Because we all have different turn-ons and diverse desires, what's sexy to you isn't necessarily what's sexy to me and vice versa. Unwashed hair, overalls, and clumsy might be a delicious combination for Mary, as very tall, rotund, and bespectacled is for Jill.

It works both ways. Not everyone we find sexy will find us sexy too. It's the luck of the draw, or chemistry, or fate, or biology, or a whole soup of mysterious things—one never knows. However, we are each sexy in our own, distinctive ways.

Here's the deal. I'm not going to tell you to look in the mirror and say affirmations that you're beautiful and sexy, or tell yourself "I love you the way you are." That may be too big a jump if you're not there yet. Continuously ask yourself, "What makes me feel confident, comfortable, grounded, joyful, connected, and mischievous?" Start noticing when you feel that way and why. Noticing these things is the first step to feeling and embracing your own brand of sexy.

If you struggle to find something nice to think or say about yourself, at least say something factual and neutral. Maybe you like your hair color or the shape of your nose. Find the parts of you that you can at least view neutrally if not positively. Return to these statements every time you notice your thinking is negative or not serving you. Soon, you will be acutely aware of how much time you spend hating on yourself, and turning your thoughts around for the better will become habit. Once you've achieved that step, keep moving forward. Admit (and believe it when you say) that "I look pretty good today." By building a practice of this kind of thinking, you will soon notice how much better you feel. You will start to gain confidence and in this way find your brand of sexy. Soon, you will be all up in your own sexiness, and there will be no stopping you!

A Little Pleasure Anatomy You May Have Missed in School

The human body is an incredible structure: It keeps us alive by operating without us having to give it much thought. Except when it comes to certain needs, our executive function (our brain) tells us what to do. When we're hungry, we eat; when we're tired, we sleep; and so on. Just like eating or sleeping, we have the option of eating for fuel or eating for pleasure, or just getting some sleep to rest our bodies or make going to sleep a relaxing and comforting ritual. Whether you treat eating or sleeping as purely a biological function or another way to enjoy your life is up to you. You decide how important these rituals are to you every day.

So it is with sexual pleasure. Sure, I can show you the positions that work best if you're a plus-size woman, but none of it will help you enjoy sex if you don't know how to perceive and extract pleasure from your own body… and I'm not just talking about orgasm. The first step to experiencing sexual pleasure is knowing how our bodies are built to give us pleasure so we can take advantage of all they have to offer!

Every Body Is Different

Each of our bodies is unique. We may all share the same basic makeup as men and women, but we certainly don't feel everything the same. What feels good on your body may not always feel good on someone else's body, and that is absolutely natural.

The skin is a person's largest organ, and we curvy gals are lucky enough to have a bit more of it. An average human body has approximately 20 square feet (1.85 square meters) of skin, with more than 200,000 nerve endings. That has potential for a lot of gratifying touching. One of the most concentrated areas of nerve endings on the female body is the head (or glans) of the clitoris, with more than 8,000 nerve endings; compare that to the head of a penis, which has about 4,000.

For every person who loves to have her feet rubbed, there is another who shudders at the thought of her feet being touched at all. Though we share the same nerve structure, the placement of those nerves in proximity to the surface of our skin can vary from person to person. Emma may love it when her partner kisses her neck—it sends shivers down her spine; Nicole may be apathetic to neck kisses but absolutely swoons when her partner kisses the inside of her wrists. The cause of this differentiation in arousable foreplay can be the culmination of many factors, but suffice it to say that we are all deliciously different. The difference between melting when your partner kisses your neck or wishing they would get to your favorite area already depends on the individual and how thick or thin her skin is and how close her nerves are to the surface.

The Vagina Is Not Your Vulva, and Vice Versa

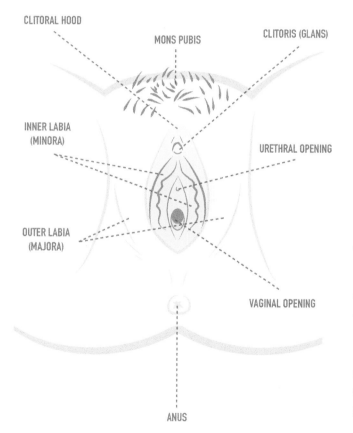

CLITORAL HOOD

MONS PUBIS

CLITORIS (GLANS)

INNER LABIA (MINORA)

URETHRAL OPENING

OUTER LABIA (MAJORA)

VAGINAL OPENING

ANUS

What's the difference between the clitoris, vulva, and the vagina? They are three different parts of your body, all with a specific purpose that can sometimes relate to each other.

The vagina is the structure *inside* the body—it is the gateway to the uterus via its doorway called the cervix. The vulva is the surrounding tissue on the *outside* of the body, guarding the vaginal opening. The vulva is made up of two sets of vaginal lips called the labia majora (outside lips) and the labia minora (inside lips). The clitoris—or rather, the outside portion of it called the glans—is located under a little "hood" of skin at the top of the inner labia, above the entrance to the vagina and the urethra, where you pee from.

It is important to remember that the vagina, vulva, and clitoris are three different structures of the body that live and work near and with each other, and each has a different job. The vagina's job is to act as the conduit for ejaculate (semen) to enter the uterus safely and potentially make a human being. The vulva's job is to protect the urethra and the vaginal opening/vagina from bacterial enemies, both foreign and domestic. And the clit—well, as far as we know, its only reason to exist is to give its owner pleasure!

These three separate parts of female genitalia all support our gynecological health, and when finding or describing what pleases you, it helps to know how each part functions.

The Clitoris is a Wishbone

What the head of the penis is to a man, the clitoris is to a woman—literally. We all start out the same in the womb until biology decides whether our erectile tissue covers a penis or is made into a nub with a set of legs and bulbs called the clitoris.

As you can see, the glans of the clit is just the tip of the proverbial iceberg. It sports a nice hood to protect it when it's not being used and is nestled in the safe, warm environment around the apex of the vulva. What you *don't* see is that extending inward, for up to 5 inches (12.7 cm) from the back of the glans, is the shaft of the clitoris. From the bottom of the glans, the shaft bends downward, bisects, and splits off into "legs" that form a shape similar to a wishbone. The clitoral legs also closely surround the vestibular bulbs directly underneath them. The vestibular bulbs are also a part of the clitoris and are attached to the shaft. When aroused, they fill with blood and hug the area around the first quarter or third of the vaginal wall. This is one of the reasons some women find the first third of their vaginal canal so pleasurable.

So don't forget that there's a whole clitoral world under the surface of your skin! By understanding that your clitoris extends inward and partly surrounds the front of your vaginal canal and outer and inner labia, you can explore how those areas feel when they are stimulated. Whether it's by yourself or with a partner, becoming familiar with the ways in which your vulva, vagina, and external and internal clitoris can be aroused can mean the difference between good sex and great sex!

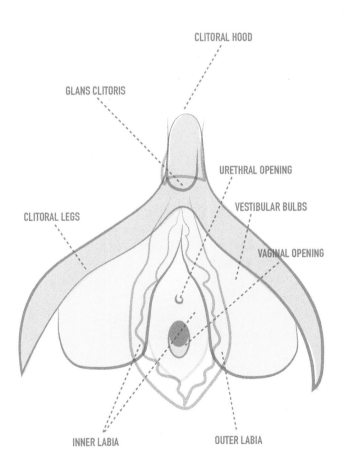

GLANS CLITORIS

CLITORAL HOOD

CLITORAL LEGS

URETHRAL OPENING

VESTIBULAR BULBS

VAGINAL OPENING

INNER LABIA

OUTER LABIA

Where Is My G-Spot?

The G-spot, which is actually more of an area than a spot, is the textured spongy area located approximately 1 to 3 inches (2.5 to 7.6 cm) inside the anterior wall of the vagina, toward your pubic bone. The G-spot is composed of erectile tissue and swells when aroused; therefore, it is easiest to find after a lot of foreplay when you are sufficiently sexually stimulated. To find it on your own, spend some time massaging your clit or vulva to get nice and aroused. Then, begin by sliding one or two fingers inside your vagina about as far as you comfortably can. Bend the fingers a bit in a "come hither" motion so that they touch the anterior wall of your vagina. You should feel a puffy patch of tissue right around there. The tissue is a little rougher than the rest, and is approximately the size of a small walnut. This is the G-spot. If you still aren't certain you've found it, spend some more time masturbating, even to the point of orgasm. Your G-spot should be fluffed up from all the excitement, making it easier to feel.

Arousal and the Importance of Foreplay

If we're to believe what we see in the movies, our sexual rendezvous would consist of 10 seconds of kissing, 5 seconds of groping, and another 5 seconds closing the deal. This just isn't realistic. A straightforward sex scene doesn't commonly show the female arousal process—and this process can sometimes take up to 40 minutes—and most of the time, this process is key in order to have a satisfying sexual experience.

Fooling around a lot before part A goes into slot B gets the female body prepped for sex in very important ways. First, the blood rushes to the vagina, engorging the vaginal canal and swelling the labia and clitoris. About the same time, your vaginal canal and the area around its entrance starts to become wet with natural lubrication, which allows for a penis, fingers, or a toy to be inserted enjoyably. If you tend to produce less lubrication than you'd like or need, reach for that bottle of lube to make insertion more comfortable. Your arousal can manifest itself in your body in other ways, as well, like nipples getting firm and more tender, skin becoming more sensitive, body temperature going up, and other senses becoming heightened.

The chief reason to engage in a lot of foreplay (other than that it's fun) is so your body has the proper time to get ready to have enjoyable sex. The next time you and your partner are in the mood and making out, extend it a bit longer than usual. Slow down and add some extra caressing, licking, eye-gazing, or gentle nibbling, then let your bodies lead you. Give yourself permission to linger in this time before you really go for it. Concentrate on enjoying the sensations you're feeling: the scent of your partner's skin, the softness of their hair, the rhythm in

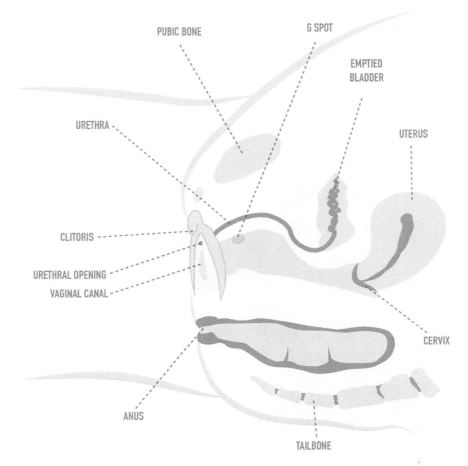

PUBIC BONE

G SPOT

EMPTIED BLADDER

URETHRA

UTERUS

CLITORIS

URETHRAL OPENING

VAGINAL CANAL

CERVIX

ANUS

TAILBONE

which you both move. Bask in the foreplay; it's one of the most enjoyable parts of sex!

I'd like to point out that, in my opinion, proper, cultivated arousal is the most important component of great sex for people with a vagina. For years, women's magazines, TV shows, and movies have been telling us that having an orgasm is the goal—the be-all and end-all of sexual pleasure. But for most women, an orgasm is just one element of the much larger pleasure picture. Lingering foreplay, sultry oral sex, sensual caressing, passionate kissing, and even just the physical feeling of penetration can rate just as highly on the pleasure scale as climaxing. In fact, for women who have

never orgasmed, or women who have a challenging time orgasming, the other delicious components of sex are vital.

Yes, orgasm can be an incredible feeling that allows you to fully take advantage of your anatomy and surrender to all the joys that can lead up to your climax. But whether you orgasm at all or you have multiple orgasms during sex, it's just part of the pleasure-filled journey—not the culmination or result.

Okay, now that you have a basic understanding of how your body is a pleasure wonderland, let's move on and look at all the accessories a voluptuous vixen can avail herself of.

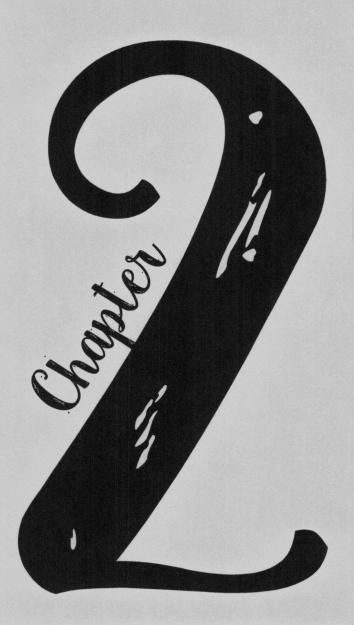

Chapter 2

Good body image is not something that most women have 24/7 . . . I think women are really selfless, and we take care of others before we take care of ourselves. Self-care rituals are really important. Whether it's working out, or how you dress, or wearing makeup, or not wearing makeup, I think all of this is really essential, and sex falls into place with that. Other people can help us feel beautiful, but they just can't do it like we can do it for ourselves.

Ducky Doolittle, sex educator
and author of *Sex with the Lights On:*
200 Illuminating Sex
Questions Answered

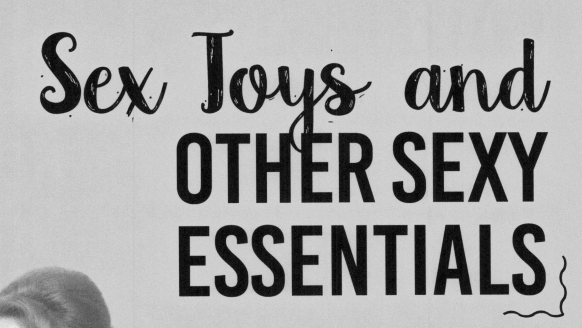

Sex Toys and OTHER SEXY ESSENTIALS

So you're ready to purchase a sex toy, but you don't know where to start. As a larger woman, it's helpful to know that there are toys that work better for your body, and even your lifestyle, by yourself and with a partner(s). First you'll want to ask yourself:

- What's your sexual lifestyle (e.g., monogamous, multiple partners, swinger)?
- What are the genders of your partners?
- Do you know the difference between a dildo and a vibrator?
- Do you prefer clit stimulation or penetration? Both? Neither?
- Do you like butt play?
- Do you like nipple massage?
- Do you enjoy BDSM (which may include intense sensations, bondage, role play, and spanking)? Or are you more drawn to candles, massage, and a fancy hotel?
- When you use your hands, how do like the pressure and speed (e.g., hard and fast, slow and soft, a combination)?
- Do you like to feel different textures or sensations on your genitals (e.g., soft and satiny, hard and prickly, electrostimulation, flogging, slapping, tickling, teasing, pinching, petting)?

The answers to these questions will help you choose the proper toys. Every woman is different, and there is an abundance of adult toys on the market to suit any desire.

Luckily, I'm very familiar with all of the options and have narrowed them down for you. In this chapter, I will detail the essential toys a curvy woman should keep next to her bed, as well a list of my all-star favorites.

Are you ready for a field trip? Take an expedition to your local sex shop. The days of the seedy storefront with cheap signs espousing XXX wares are mostly behind us. Now, gentrified, female-friendly shops exist in most major cities (e.g., The Pleasure Chest, Good Vibrations, Babeland, Smitten Kitten). Browse the merchandise. You don't need to be shy, because everyone is there for the same reason and the staff has heard and seen it all. Let yourself drift into that part of you that is adventurous and craves touch and pleasure. Your instinct won't lead you astray!

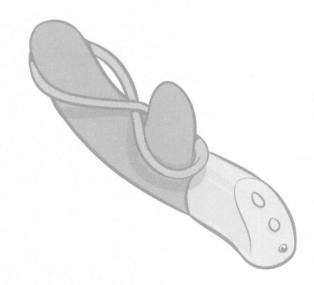

WHAT IS A BODY-SAFE SEX TOY?

Call me crazy, but if I'm putting something in my body, I want to know that it doesn't contain toxic materials. Sex toys are not regulated by the government, so when you're shopping for a sex toy that goes in your body, you might want to steer clear of certain ingredients like phthalates, polyvinyl chloride (PVC), "jelly" rubber, or vinyl. Some studies suggest that continued exposure to these chemicals might lead to cancer. Even some nontoxic toys can still be porous, meaning they can harbor bacteria in tiny crevices that are almost impossible to completely sanitize. If you buy or already have a toy and aren't certain whether it's toxic or porous, don't fret! Just put an unlubricated condom on it when you're ready to use it, and you're good to go!

Regardless of what types of toys you're using, *always* clean your toys after each use. Specialty toy cleaner, or even regular soap and hot water, can prevent an unpleasant infection.

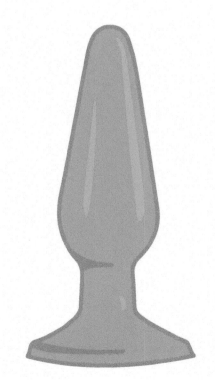

Lube: You Can't Get Enough

A common misconception among men and women alike is that personal lubricant exists only for the chronically dry vagina and butt sex. While lube may be essential in those two instances, it is by no means the only time lube should be used. So how often should you use lube? All the time! What are the scenarios that call for lube? All scenarios! Radical concept? Not really, and I'll tell you why.

First of all, the viscosity, abundance, and ability to produce our natural secretions can be affected by so many different factors—from our exercise level and where we are in our cycle to medication side effects and even stress. These reasons, plus the fact that our natural juices wax and wane throughout an interlude with our partner (or ourselves), are reason enough to keep lube on your nightstand.

> "The term sexual wellness means being able to embrace one's sexuality and fully enjoy the act of sex. Research has shown that women who use lubricant actually have higher levels of sexual satisfaction and pleasure, and experience less pain during intercourse. Not only does lubricant prevent vaginal tearing and keep condoms from tearing, it also enhances the sexual experience for both women and their partners. It aids in both sexual health and wellness, and helps people enjoy sex more."
>
> **—Dr. Emily Morse, sexologist, author, and host of _Sex with Emily_**

But did you know that using lubricant is also just good hygiene? Using lube helps to prevent micro-tears on the delicate skin in and on the genitals, which leave us more vulnerable to sexually transmitted infections. Lube also makes the friction between your vagina (or anus) and whatever is being inserted silky and comfortable, and also assists in smooth and nongrating hand sex. Using lube has been known to make penetrative sex last longer, and also even a drop in the well of a condom can make wearing one a lot more comfy. In fact, using a water-based lube with a toy during solo sex makes for more delightful contact and, because of the conductive qualities of liquids and gels, can possibly enhance a good vibration. Trust me, you need and want lube in your nightstand.

Convinced? Good. Now you need to know there are four kinds of lubricants (sometimes called "glides") that you may come across on your lube hunt: water-based, silicone, hybrid, and oil. Generally, oil-based lubes are not recommended for vaginal penetration, because oil can make for a breeding ground for bacteria and cause an infection. The exception to this is coconut oil, which has some naturally occurring antibacterial properties and may be more resistant to the bacteria that causes vaginal infections. Also, it's important to note that most commercial lubes that you're likely to find at the supermarket or drugstore could contain ingredients like parabens, polypropylene glycol, and glycerin, which can irritate some vaginas. To play it safe, I always recommend getting a premium lube that has as few ingredients as possible. Read carefully, because some lubes can be used only under certain conditions. Also, if you like to use earth-friendly, organic, or vegan products, you're in luck! There are a few brands that fit that bill, but my favorite is Sliquid. Check the resources at the back of this book for more suggestions.

Lube Options

LUBE TYPE	PROS	CONS
Water-based lube	The most versatile; can be used on all sex toys and condoms. Can also come flavored. Condom safe.	May not last as long.
Silicone lube	Long lasting. Typically hypoallergenic. Very slippery (great for hand jobs, masturbation, and long sex sessions with your partner). Condom safe.	Not to be used with silicone toys.
Hybrid (water-based lube with some silicone)	More slippery than water-based lube. Lasts longer than water-based lube. Can usually be used with silicone toys (but check the label of the product you want to use it with). Condom safe. Less slippery than silicone.	Doesn't last as long as silicone
Coconut oil*	Long-lasting, very slippery, natural.	Do not use with condoms.

*Generally, oil-based lubes are not recommended for vaginal penetration because they can create a breeding ground for bacteria and cause an infection. The exception to this is coconut oil, which has some naturally occurring antibacterial properties and may be more resistant to causing vaginal infections.

Silicone Lube: It's Not Just for Sex Anymore

Silicon lube is the gift that keeps on giving! You can use premium silicone lube for other personal uses too, such as:

- Work a drop into your hair as a gloss.
- Rub it on your inner thighs to avoid chafing.
- Use it as a makeshift shaving oil when shaving your legs.
- Apply it sparingly as a body moisturizer.
- Apply a drop to your face as a makeup primer.
- Use it to take off a sticky price tag.

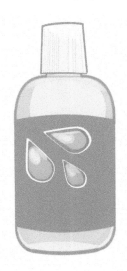

The Best Vibrators for Curvy Girls

Vibrators can be designed for external stimulation, penetration, or both. If you are like many women and you need clitoral stimulation to orgasm, you might want to have one or two of these puppies handy. If clitoral stimulation isn't your jam, these vibes can still be enjoyable on any erogenous zone, like nipples, taint (perineum), inside the butt cheeks (but outside the anus), or at the top of your mons. You never know until you try, and trying is half the fun!

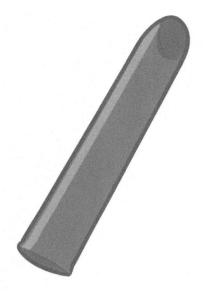

Bullet Vibrator

A bullet vibrator should be a staple in your bedside arsenal because of its size and the power it packs. Small, thin, fat, long, short—these vibes come in a variety of sizes, but they're typically shaped like a bullet. Bullets are great alone, used in concert with a harness, or used by your partner to stimulate your clit while he or she otherwise occupies your vagina. A common way to use a bullet vibe is when your bodies are pressed together, such as in the missionary position, where the pressure between your bodies holds the bullet vibe in place. There are a million of these on the market and the price range is vast, but I suggest investing in a rechargeable, body-safe bullet vibe with a variety of strengths and settings, such as the WeVibe Tango or Touch. However, if you're not certain a bullet is for you and you want something inexpensive to try before you invest, the Screaming O makes a variety of bullet vibes at affordable prices. Some are even disguised as lipsticks or mascara in case you're traveling incognito.

Wand Vibrator

Wand vibrators have a long handle with a "head" at one end that creates a very strong vibration. Wands (or "massagers," as they were called back in the day) were originally developed to give people extra reach and range of motion to massage aching neck and back muscles. It didn't take long before women discovered that the vibrations from the wands worked wonders between their legs! For the curvy gal, a wand is key. Because of its length and strength, a wand can navigate over a large stomach to reach the clit with ease. Another reason a wand is a fantastic tool to keep close is that women with big tummies can tuck the handle of the wand under their soft belly to hold it in place during missionary-style sex.

The most well-known toy in the wand category, the Original Magic Wand is the massager that started it all in the '70s and is still a bestseller today, especially among women who like intense vibration.

A Massager Wand by Doxy also offers strong, more rumbly vibration. If you like less intensity, try a smaller wand by Vibratex called the Mystic Wand. Tantus had people with reach issues in mind when designing the Rumble vibrator, as it has a slight curve and a flexible head, and offers different head attachments. There are other companies that make wands of various strengths and lengths that are also terrific. See Curvy Resources, page 178, for more choices.

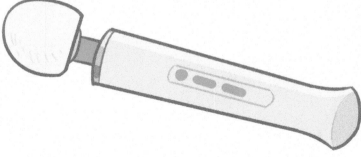

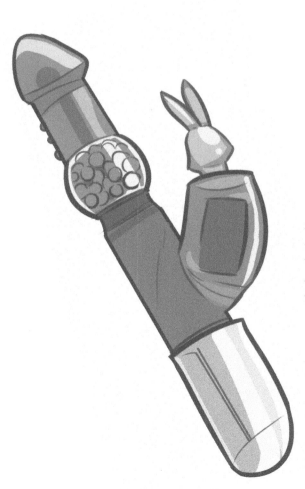

Rabbit Vibrator

You might have heard of this well-known style of vibe from friends or whispers on the subway, or you may have even seen it on *Sex and the City*. The rabbit-style vibrator is both a vibrating dildo and a clitoral stimulator that can act in concert with each other or separately. The rabbit vibe is shaped like a phallus, with a little rabbit head and ears poking out at the base of the shaft, just before the handle. There are traditionally two sets of controls on the rabbit vibe's handle: one vibrates the shaft to stimulate the vaginal walls, and the other vibrates the ears to stimulate the clitoris. Because of its dual-stimulation capability, this type of vibe is a bestseller online and in adult shops worldwide. However, maneuvering a linear object over curves and at an angle can be a Herculean task. Thank goodness for the Joystick by Vibratex. Originally made as an ergonomic choice to please women with carpal tunnel syndrome, this rabbit vibrator is curved at about a 110-degree angle, making it easier to navigate voluptuous tummies. How genius is that?

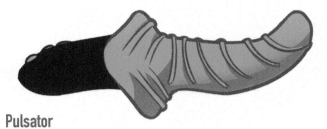

Pulsator

Not everyone who wants vibration is interested in direct clitoral stimulation; for some women, that can actually be painful. Some bodies prefer vaginal vibration to arouse them and make them climax. The majority of vibrators use a motor to create different levels and patterns of vibration. However, there is a new category of vibrators called pulsators. Pulsators are self-propelled dildos that can be used hands-free. After insertion in the vagina (using water-based lube, please), the pulsator literally moves back and forth with some impressive strength. The end result is a motorized dildo that penetrates the vagina (or anus, if you like) and plunges in and out, mimicking partner intercourse with a penis or dildo. Fun Factory is the only company that currently makes pulsators. Luckily, it includes a set of instructions for use with every device. I've found that, regardless of size, placing a pillow between your legs to keep the pulsator from flying across the room (and traumatizing the dog for life) is a smart move. Not only does that relieve you from holding it in place, but it also allows you to lay back and fantasize while the pulsator has its way with you.

G-Spotter

Sometimes called a Slimline vibe for its telltale width, the Slimline is simply shaped like a rod with a bent bulbous tip. These vibes are usually affordable, battery operated, and come in a variety of lengths from 5 to 10 inches (12.7 to 25.4 cm) long. The Slimline is an excellent tool for discovering and becoming familiar with your G-spot. Curvy girls love it for the length, as it's pretty easy to maneuver and can also be used on the clit like a bullet with a long handle. Think of it kind of like a selfie stick for your clit!

The Best Dildos for Curvy Girls

If you like that feeling of fullness inside you when you're aroused or if you can orgasm from penetration (with or without clitoral stimulation), you'll want to explore the wonderful world of dildos. Dildos (sometimes called insertables) can be made from many different materials, including ceramic, plastic, wood, steel, stone, glass, and elastomer. However, the most commonly enjoyed dildos are made from high-quality, body-safe silicone. Personally, I suggest staying away from highly porous materials like jelly, rubber, PVC, and cyberskin/RealSkin/UR3, which may contain ingredients (such as phthalates) that are considered less safe for the body. Trusted sex blogs like the Redhead Bedhead, Hey Epiphora, and Dangerous Lilly will help you learn more about materials and give you expert reviews.

This is an area where shape, size, and materials can really matter for any shapely woman. When shopping for a dildo, you'll want to consider length, curve, and bendability. If you're interested in a little more adaptability, there are companies that make body-safe dildos with a suction-cup base that can temporarily attach to most surfaces, like a shower wall, a floor, or even a refrigerator. Some dildos come with a removable bullet vibe to add vibration. If you've already purchased a sturdy, well-made bullet vibe of your own, you may want to try using it instead of the bullet vibes that come with the dildo (which tend to be weaker or not last as long).

The dildo shapes, models, and brands that I most commonly recommend for curvy girls are on this page and the next; however, in most cases, the dildo's shape and intended use is more important than brand.

Dildo with Handle

Tantus is the only company I've found that makes silicone dildos with handles, which it added to some of its most popular models so people of size and some people with mobility issues would be able to enjoy them. The handle models come in four shapes, with insertable lengths that vary from 6.5 to 10 inches (16.5 to 25.4 cm) and widths that vary as well. The handles of these premium dildos gradually morph into a bendable shaft, which ranges in diameter and texture to suit your fancy. Though these aren't made for harness use, the handle and length, coupled with a firm yet flexible shaft, make these dildos a staple for your nightstand.

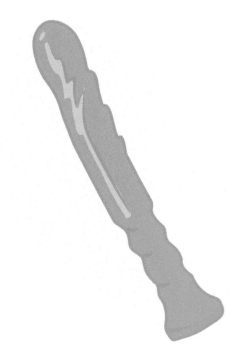

Heavy Metal

Okay, I know it's may sound strange, but if you like having your G-spot stimulated, or are just curious to find out if you do, this stainless-steel dildo could become your favorite toy.

The Njoy Pure Wand is 1½ pounds (0.6 kg) and 8½ inches (21.6 cm) of smooth, nonporous, shiny medical-grade stainless steel. The Pure Wand has a large and a small bulb on either end to inspire arousal in the G-spot. For some, this is the vehicle by which they've discovered the potential of their G-spot, and sometimes even female ejaculation. For others, it's just cool, weighty, insertable fun. The heft of the stainless steel gives the user greater control over the pressure exerted while using it, and the unique curve is such that it can navigate larger tummies or thighs—and, if you enjoy anal play, the booty. I don't know a single sex educator that doesn't own one of these beauties.

Large and in Charge

Want a little more girth in your phallus? Looking for something a little more representational? Then have I got a dick for you! The Mason by New York Toy Collective is 8 inches (20.3 cm) of dual-density (squishy on the outside with a firm inner core), bendable soft silicone. This dildo is soft and pliable to the touch, and yet can bend a bit in order to get to all the hard-to-reach places. It can be used in a harness for some strap-on fun, and because it has a wide-enough base, it can be used for anal play as well... if you dare.

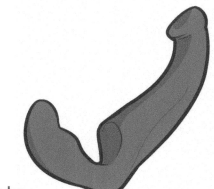

The Double Header

Double-ended dildos have come a long way since the neon, yard-long jelly dongs of yore. Nowadays they are more ergonomic, comfortable, and versatile and can be used myriad ways. Take the modern double-ended dildos like the Fun Factory Share or Tantus FeelDoe, for example. These dildos are a gem for the curvy gal. Usually about 10 inches (25.4 cm) long and made to be worn as a "strapless strap-on," these toys have a shape that resembles an L. One end is a short dildo that the giver can insert and secure by clenching with her pubococcygeal (PC) muscles while she penetrates the receiver with the longer end. Curvy gals might also love this dildo for solo use, holding one end as a handle while penetrating themselves with the other end. The shape also lends itself to solo sex in different positions—like doggy-style, missionary, standing up, or lying on one's side—because it can be long and flexible enough to work with and around curves. Another plus? These models are sometimes offered with a vibrating option using a removable bullet vibe. Whatever option you decide, a double-ended, wearable dildo is a no-brainer for women who love the feeling of fullness that penetration provides.

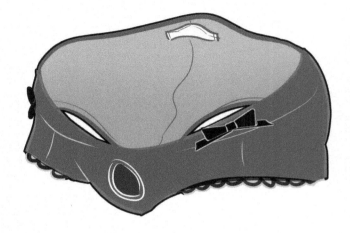

Other Accessories

Sometimes what we want to do requires a little extra help, and this is when harnesses, straps, and sex furniture are nice to have around.

Harnesses

If you think it's hard to find cool lingerie and clothes in your size, try looking for a harness for strap-on play. It's not easy, but I found some that are not only well-made but beautiful and comfortable to wear.

SpareParts makes harnesses up to a size 5X US/32 UK/34 AUS. Some have lace, some have ruching and garters, and some are just classic and simple, but what they all have in common is that they are incredibly comfortable and look terrific on a curvy body. Sportsheets International has a plus-size line of harnesses that are budget-friendly and work great, and Tantus has its simple but serviceable Vibrating Velvet Harness. Each of these models has a secret pocket inside the front panel of the harness to fit a vibrating bullet, so there's a little something in it for both of you.

Harness Hacks

- If you have a harness with nylon webbing straps that's a little snug and could use some extra length, you can purchase a "harness extender" or pop into a camping or Army/Navy store and pick up some extra nylon webbing in the length you need and switch it out when you get home.

- Try wearing the harness without a dildo and with the bullet vibe in the pocket for hands-free solo fun! With a slight adjustment, you can pull the front panel of the harness (the part that holds the bullet vibe) down so that it rests on top of your mons or clit

Straps

The Doggy Style Strap is a long piece of nylon webbing with a padded panel in the middle. On each end of the webbing, there is a loop to use as a handle. The idea is that the strap is positioned underneath the receiver's hips and around the lower abdomen when she is in the doggy-style position (on her hands and knees) and the giver, to aid in penetrating the receiver, holds on to the straps using the loops at each end and pulls the receiver back toward him as he thrusts. This is a fun and functional accessory if you have weaker back or arms, as the giver and strap act as a support, taking weight off of the receiver and, of course, providing deeper (and if you like, more forceful) penetration. Plus-size versions of this strap are available, or you can use the Liberator Slingshot as the doggy-style strap by having the giver use the cuffs as handles, or wrapping excess nylon webbing around his hands until the desired length is achieved.

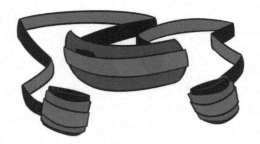

Liberator Wedge

For any of the positions in this book that I suggest using pillows for, I recommend using a Liberator Wedge instead. The Liberator Wedge (and the other sizes and shapes they make) is fashioned out of industrial foam and has a removable, washable cover. The industrial foam doesn't have much give, so it doesn't squash down to a pancake when you put weight on it like a pillow can. A Wedge placed under the butt not only raises it higher to make oneself more open and available for one's partner but it also uses gravity to its advantage where copious bellies are concerned. Because of the downward slope the torso has while resting on the Wedge, anything in the midsection that jiggles will flow away from the genital area making access even easier for the giver and for any hands that want to stimulate the clit. Speaking of which, the Wedge is genius for oral or hand sex: it raises the vulva to meet the giver's mouth, again pulling the tummy back and away from the hips, clearing the way for some major grazing.

Sex Starter Kit

If you have a nightstand with drawers, devote one drawer to all your sexy essentials such as sex toys, lube, condoms, blindfolds, and, of course, this book. Keep designated, firm pillows in a nearby closet or under the bed so you don't have to search for them should they come in handy for some of your positions. The same goes for small towels or washcloths. Sex is messy at best, so why not have a few towels assigned for clean-up at the ready? Finally, sex is a workout, so keep glasses or bottles of water nearby for you and for your partner to rehydrate before round two.

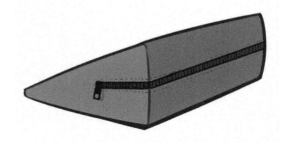

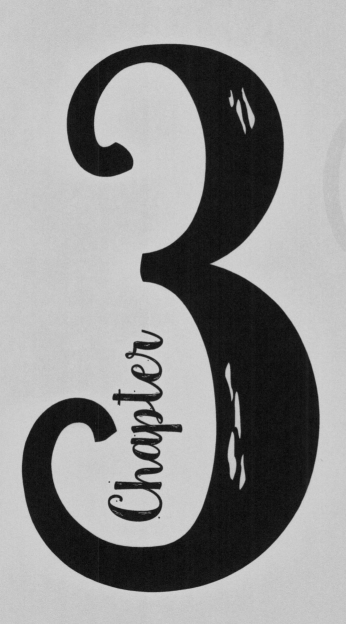

Chapter 3

One of the most powerful things to do if you're having body image issues is to see yourself eroticized and sexualized . . . to have that reflected back is really powerful and healing.

Chris Donaghue, Ph.D., author of *Sex Outside the Lines* **and cohost of** *LoveLine*

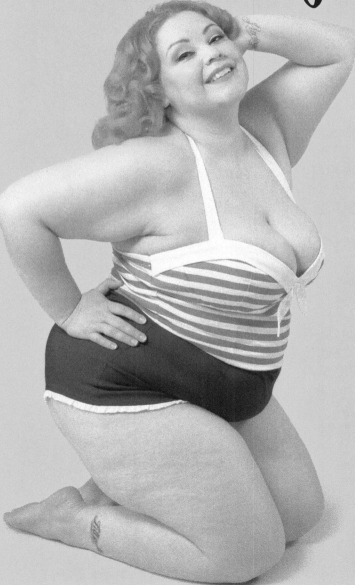

Curvy Girl prep:

SENSUALITY, COMMUNICATION, AND GETTING IN THE MOOD

When it comes to getting down, I like to look at sex like food, and sensuality is its flavor.

Like food, sex can be satiating. It feeds our hunger and nourishes our body—you might even argue we need it to live. But if you think about it, making food delicious to eat and crave-worthy relies on flavor (and technique). The flavor is unique to the chef preparing the food and then interpreted by the palate of the taster. A food's flavor can be simple, it can be sweet or spicy, or it can open up a variety of senses. Sensuality is similar. Everyone is his or her own chef—attracting diners who crave their dishes.

Often, we ignore sensual opportunities to make room for other day-to-day needs, like grabbing a sandwich on the way home from work because you're too tired to make dinner. But would you skip a nap or your morning coffee if you've been losing sleep? Prioritizing your sensuality and unifying it with your sexual self commands just as much of your attention. Allow yourself to become aware of your senses and what makes you feel sexy, turns you on, and feels good against your skin. Notice what music excites you, what smells make you feel serene, and what food you crave. These are gateways to discovering your particular brand of sensuality.

Owning our sexiness builds confidence and encourages boldness in our everyday lives. When you feel sensual, you are better able to feel sexy. And when you feel sexy, you're feeling positive—and I think we can all agree that feeling positive makes a huge difference in our daily lives. So what do you have to lose?

Embrace the Senses

Consider each of your five senses and evaluate how you tend to engage them. For example, what do you like to feel against your skin?

- What's the texture? Is it rough? Soft? Smooth?
- Is it wet or dry?
- How does it make you feel? Does it change your mood?
- Does it give you comfort or make you feel sexy?

If you ask yourself these types of questions about each sense, you'll better understand what elicits a sensual response for you. Then, you can better integrate those senses and feelings into your everyday life.

Wear that sexy underwear to work, pack strawberries in your lunch, and enjoy sultry music during your day. Embrace this newfound awareness, and make it a part of your daily ritual. It seems elementary, but you will be surprised how sexy you will feel when you least expect to. You don't have to act on it; you just have to feel it. You might even recognize that you feel a bit more confident and that the people around you are responding to that. Good work!

The more you explore, the more natural you will feel expressing yourself. This is essential whether you are partnered or single. The more comfortable you are with your own sensuality and sexuality, the more confident you will be in the bedroom. Figuring out what makes you feel sexy helps fuel the romance when you meet someone you want to be intimate with.

Alone Time

Indulge your inner sex kitten and set aside some quality time alone to explore and get to know how your body likes to be touched. For some, bedtime is a good choice, and for others first thing in the morning is more appealing. Wherever you are, make certain the room is conducive to getting turned on. Soft lighting, music, silky sheets, whatever floats your boat—set up your atmosphere in a way that makes you feel sensual and delicious. Prepare for an intimate date night with yourself.

Respect the time you've set aside for sexual pleasure, and make certain you don't inadvertently set yourself up to fail. If you're anxiously awaiting a call from work in an hour, chances are you won't be able to fully relax into your body and be present. Turn off phones, put pets in another room, and make sure no one will be able to disturb you. Get naked and into whatever position is comfortable and feels organic. Above all, honor this time.

Start to explore your body with your hands and fingers. Run your fingertips over every part of your body, at first very slowly, and then do it again with various speeds and levels of pressure. Follow your instinct and let your fingers take you wherever they want to go. Perhaps begin with the parts of your body that yearn for a soft graze or a warm hand.

Sometimes people can experience judgmental thoughts, or feelings of embarrassment or shame. If this happens to you, just acknowledge that you're having that thought, and then gently bring your attention back to your fingers and hands on your skin. Regardless, the goal here is not to orgasm but to tune into your body, and where and how it likes to be touched.

When you notice a particular spot that feels better than the rest, linger there and explore. Sometimes the most surprising spot can be titilating. When you make your way to your nipples, vulva, vagina, and clit, notice how you're touching yourself.

- How fast or slow are you going? Does your speed build or decrease throughout, or does it vary?
- Do you like light touch, pressure, or no touch at all?
- Do you like your labial lips massage, stroked, grazed?
- Do you like fingers inside your vagina?
- Are your breasts more sensitive than your clit? How do you like them touched? Do you like to stimulate them at the same time as your clit?

Sensuality is all about your own personal path to pleasure, the courage to explore it, and the confidence that comes from understanding that part of you. Knowing what makes us feel sensual and sexy is an important tool for sexual self-confidence. At the end of the day, this time is an investment in your sex life. What a fun assignment! When you carve out time to discover all the different ways you like to be aroused, you are armed with that information and better able to show your partner what gets you going.

Erotica: Not Your Mother's Romance Novel

Some people use erotica to get in a seductive mood and coax their sensual self to the surface. Today's erotica is adventurous, explicit, and *very* hot. Reading another's account of sexual exploits, true or imagined, can be empowering and exhilarating, and reinforces how natural and rich our own sensuality is.

We all know the stereotype of the paperback romance novel, with the dramatic cover art of a muscled, tan, and long-haired scoundrel of a man catching a voluptuous, raven-haired beauty in his strong, capable arms. Times have changed, and with it, the available options of literary excitement. Erotic novels and short stories have become the go-to for racy, sexed-up romps of lust, love, and kink.

You're likely familiar with *Fifty Shades of Grey*, but I'm happy to share that there are plenty more well-established modern erotica authors and anthologists turning out lusty novels, stories, and compilations created for all genders, sexualities, fetishes, kinks, body types, relationship models, and more. Look for works by Rachel Kramer Bussel, Kristina Wright, Tristan Taormino, and Violet Blue, just to name a few.

If you're a literary buff or you prefer your erotica vintage, you can find steamy and passionate love stories in books or correspondence between famous lovers like Anaïs Nin and Henry Miller, John Keats and Fanny Brawne, or Jean-Paul Sartre and Simone de Beauvoir. Or check out the sensual love (and lust) poetry of Pablo Neruda, e.e. Cummings, Charles Bukowski, or 13th-century poet and scholar Rumi. There's even fantasy erotica, like A. N.

Roquelaure's Sleeping Beauty series or Charlaine Harris's Sookie Stackhouse series, which was turned into the hit HBO series *True Blood*.

There's erotica to suit everyone's taste. So consider what kind of dynamic, era, or style you want to get you going, then visit your local bookstore or discreetly download those titles online.

Feminist Porn: It Exists and It's Awesome

When Candida Royalle started making porn for women in 1984, she created an international appetite for explicit adult entertainment that wasn't created solely for male, heterosexual pleasure. Sometimes called feminist porn or couples porn, these movies focus more on sensuality, desire, passion, and women's pleasure, as opposed to the more mainstream porn that started the adult entertainment industry. Today, this genre has exploded to include "beautiful porn," feminist porn, and queer porn. Trailblazers in this category include feminist female filmmakers like Tristan Taormino and Erika Lust, who make certain that their actors are treated fairly and respectfully. They create sexy, sensual visuals and storylines, and always make certain their actors have chemistry, connection, and real orgasms.

Feminist porn is also more body-positive. These films are often shot without regard to how thin or fit the actors are. In fact, many feminist porn production companies pride themselves on featuring varied body types and sizes without fetishizing those bodies. These production companies are becoming more and more popular, especially with women who want to see actors on-screen who look more like they do.

The New Porn: Bite-size and Empowering

Lots of Internet sites deliver short-form porn, which I call *new porn*. New porn is blogger-selected sex scenes cut to a-few-seconds-long clips called gifs and intermingled with erotic photography. New porn is handy if you want to get aroused and then get off without committing to a 90-minute movie.

Tumblr.com is one of the best places to find new porn. Tumblr is a free social media and blogging platform well known for its many user-curated erotica/porn blogs (including my own, www.LadyCheeky.com). To find and discover the kind of arousing eye candy that appeals to you on Tumblr, use search terms like "sexy," "passion," "making love," or "kissing." Or sign up for a free account and widen the vocabulary you can use to search for terms and perhaps create and curate your own Tumblr porn site. Use your own Tumblr photo blog with a partner or lover as a means of communicating or negotiating the sexual activities you each want (or don't want) to try. Some use these sites as ways to get turned on with their partner, especially in a long-distance relationship or with a partner who travels frequently. For more suggestions on erotic porn sites and other Internet resources, check out my list at the back of this book.

Use Your Words

You might want to begin the conversation by telling your partner about something that he or she does (or you do together) sexually that you really like, and then suggest a new idea. For instance, "I've been thinking about how exciting it is when you give me a little swat on my butt during sex," then add, "I think I'd like it if you tug at my hair a bit, too." During sex can also be great time to show your lover that you appreciate what he's doing. A well-placed "Yes, just like that" or a simple "Oh, yes!" will guide him in the right direction. Don't be shy to express your pleasure. I guarantee this positive reinforcement will not only turn your partner on but will give him or her a more specific map of your pleasure zones.

Direct the Scene

Sometimes you have to physically show your partner what you need. For example, if you'd like your partner to stroke your hair when he kisses you, take his hand and direct it in the way that pleases you. Offer approving glances and sounds as he follows your lead. It goes without saying that your positive reinforcement when he successfully mimics your movements will be all the affirmation he needs to happily continue.

Cybersex

If social media has taught us one thing, it's that anonymity can erase our inhibitions and allow us to say things we may not have the courage to say in person. Whether you've just started flirting with someone online or your partner is away on a trip, cybersex can be a fun way to explore your turn-ons—and those of your partner. When communicating this way with someone you don't know and trust, and *especially* if you use your camera, be careful about how much personal information and identifying traits you reveal. It's not difficult for someone to record and share that information.

Fantasy: Exploring Your Sexual Desires

Fantasies are a large part of a healthy sex life. Respecting and expressing your own needs in a responsible and loving way builds your sexual confidence. Never forget that *you* are in charge of your own sexuality, and you deserve an exciting, sensual, and communicative sex life!

Suggestive Role-Play

If the idea of role-playing gets your juices flowing, start with something fun and sexy you two can chuckle about later. Maybe your partner has a thing for uniforms? Surprise her by donning a few key items from a professional's gear. Become a first responder and sport a firefighter's hat. Don't be afraid to be goofy. Goofy can be fun (and sexy) and nothing relaxes people more than a good-natured laugh. Suggest that next time your partner might play a Navy lieutenant and "rescue" you from the enemy. You've embraced your lighthearted side, shown her your fantasy, and communicated your desires without needing a serious conversation!

Take a Walk on the Lighter Side

Interested in trying Tantra but dreading your partner's eye roll because of its woo-woo reputation? Structured breathing is at the core of Tantra—and what could be more natural and normal than breathing? Look up some simple Tantric breathing exercises and choose one that works for you. In fact, you might suggest to your partner that you perform a Tantric exercise before foreplay to "get in the zone." My favorite resource for breathing exercises and Tantra is *Urban Tantra* by Barbara Carrellas. Barbara also has a really informative website (www.barbaracarrellas. com), with free downloadable exercises and worksheets to help you foster more intimate communication and get in the mood. By easing an idea into your routine, you just might be surprised at how eager your partner is to please and happy to oblige.

Getting The Kinks Out

Always fantasized about dabbling in your dark side? Nervous about how to bring it up to your partner? Try introducing kink by reading aloud some kinky erotica! Prolific erotica authors Rachel Kramer Bussel and Tristan Taormino have a lot to choose from. Or if you want to start with something closer to *Fifty Shades of Grey*, in the throes of passion, try holding your partner's hands over her head while you're on top. Maybe whip out a silky sleep mask before you introduce the idea of a blindfold. The key is to start slow and arm yourself with knowledge of how to play sexy and safe.

Talking Dirty Is Good Clean Fun

Some people believe that dirty talk is only for specific occasions when the pace is fast and furious and both of you can't get your clothes off quickly enough. However, there is a very good reason to engage in talking dirty when having sex, and that has everything to do with encouraging good communication. In fact, people have had aural sex for a millennia—where do you think we got all our best curse words from?

In school, many of us learned the "famous six" when we were taught the proper way to write a story. In a story, you need to know the what, who, where, why, when, and how. If starting the smut-speak stumps you, start there. Think about *what* you would like, *where* you would like it, *why* you want it, *when* it needs to happen, and *how* you want it done. For example, you might say, "I'm craving your cock in my mouth right now. I want you to come in my mouth." Once you have the famous six down pat, get creative and throw in some adjectives. For example, "My mouth is hungry for your delicious cock. I want you to come in it, hard."

Besides being great for sharing your desires, dirty talk can serve a greater purpose—keeping you focused in the moment. Dirty talk facilitates being and staying present when you are with your partner. You can't be worrying about the electric bill (or your tummy) while you're uttering, "That's it baby, rub it faster. Fuck me with your tongue." Making a commitment to being present when you're in bed lays a perfect foundation for developing sexual intimacy and for building trust and heat with your lover. When you're in bed with someone and you're thinking about the laundry, a conference call the next day, or if he or she thinks your ass is too big, you're not connecting with your partner; you're giving less of yourself and by extension giving less to your lover.

Intention is everything. If you're distracted, it translates to how you're touching your partner and how he or she is receiving your touch, and you're likely not taking the most pleasure from your time together. But if you're stroking your partner and telling her, explicitly, how good she feels ("It turns me on how wet your pussy is"), how you like the way he's moving to your rhythm ("That's right, baby, fuck my hands with your cock"), how beautiful or handsome they look ("I love the way you look when you're turned on"), or how hot she is ("Fuck, you're so sexy—I want to consume you") your attention is on your partner, and not only does your partner feel it, but your observations add to your own arousal and the sexual energy you are creating together.

Reframing a question in a sexy way as part of seduction/foreplay allows couples to be clear about what kind of sexual activity is allowed while keeping the mood alive. Saying, "I'd really like to be inside you right now," or "I'm wondering what it would be like to kiss you" in a soft, seductive tone can feel easier (and hotter) in a steamy moment than, "Would you like to have sex?" or "Do you mind if I kiss you?" Answering the question can work the same way. For example, you might respond, "Yes, yes, put it inside me," or if you'd rather not, "Mmm, I'd rather keep kissing your soft lips." This kind of consent communication keeps the permission ongoing and clear (and hopefully enthusiastic), while still maintaining an erotic atmosphere. It's a good idea to be aware of the general mood of the moment. If you're feeling any unstated apprehension from your partner, better to check in and ask how she's feeling. When you and your lover both clearly understand exactly what is being asked for, it takes a whole lot of pressure off both of you.

"Think of some words to describe bodies: 'big,' 'strong,' 'soft,' 'zaftig,' 'curvaceous,' 'voluptuous.' These words can be worshipful, arousing, and loving, as in, 'Sit that gorgeous big ass on my face,' or 'You're so strong! Hold me down with those huge arms!' or 'I love holding your soft belly in my hands when I fuck you from behind.' But those words can also remind us that the world is unkind to us about our bodies, which is not a sexy or empowering association. The best way to create pleasure and satisfaction from this confusion is to understand what specific erotic language means to you and how it makes you feel."

Tina Horn, author of *Sexting*

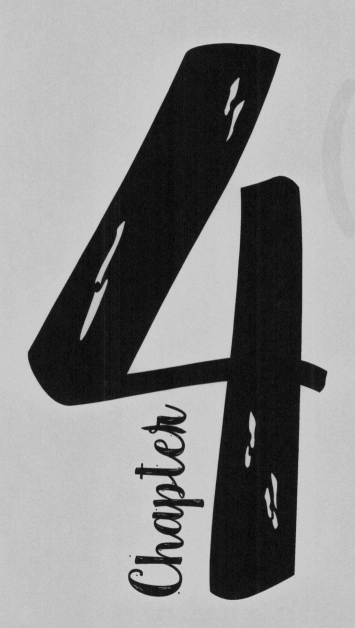

Chapter

4

Masturbation is a meditation on self-love. So many of us are afflicted with self-loathing, bad body images, shame about our body functions, and confusion about sex and pleasure; I recommend an intense love affair with yourself.

**Betty Dodson, Ph.D., sexologist
and author of *Sex for One***

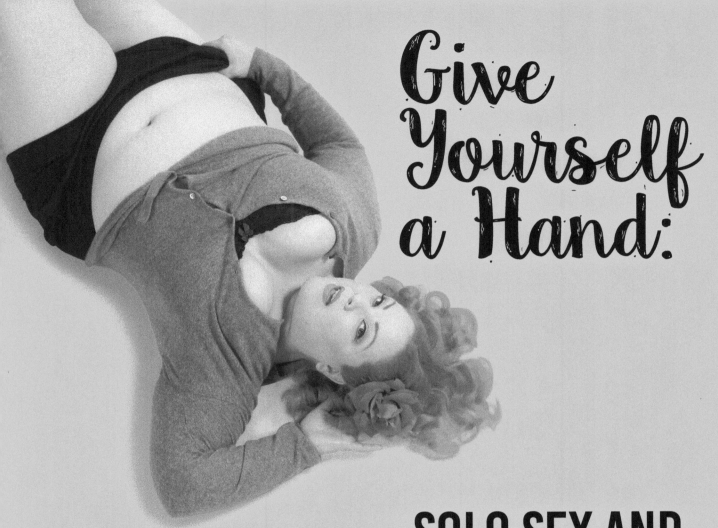

Give Yourself a Hand:

SOLO SEX AND THE IMPORTANCE OF SELF-PLEASURE

Knowing how you like to be touched and being able to communicate that kindly to a partner is a major component of a satisfying sex life.

But how do you know what makes your body sing if you haven't spent some time finding out? Solo sex is a natural way to understand what *your* particular body likes and how it likes to be aroused.

Solo sex has a bunch of other benefits, too. For instance, some women swear that an orgasm helps them fall asleep easily. Women with menstrual cramps have reported that having an orgasm helps alleviate the pain, and of course it's the perfect remedy to sate your sex drive when you're feeling especially amorous. Another great reason to get yourself off regularly is that it exercises your sexual side and helps you feel sexy. It awakens the part of you that that is kept at bay most of the time and allows it to express itself. Also, for this particular book, having solo sex regularly is part of staying connected to your body, feeling sensual, and acknowledging that your sexuality has nothing to do with body size or shape, but everything to do with being human and experiencing pleasure.

Whether solo sex is an occasional pastime, or if you're a masturbation maven, grab a bottle of lube, sit back, and enjoy the following positions, tips, and tricks for curvy gals who self-explore.

Solo Fifth Position

Perhaps the most traditional of all self-love poses, "on the back" is commonly one of the first positions women try when starting to self-stimulate. If you prefer your self-loving on your back, but your back isn't into it, spread your legs, bend your knees, and bring the soles of your feet together. This separates the thighs and opens up the labial folds, making self-stimulation easy and breezy.

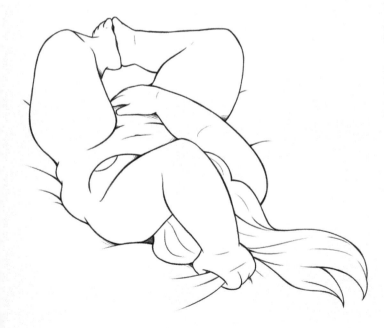

From Badgering the Witness to Roughing Up the Suspect

When it comes to masturbation, we're probably all familiar with at least a couple of slang terms to describe it (e.g., jack off, rub one out, fap). But did you know that there are more than 500 unique idioms for solo sex? It's true! Here are some of my favorites that you might want to consider adding to your lascivious lexicon:

Airing out the orchid

Pearl diving/pearl fishing

Feeding the bearded clam

Hitchhiking south

Paddling the pink canoe

Playing the clitar

Tiptoeing through the two-lips

Trolling the Bermuda Triangle

Pushing the button

Voting for the clit commander

Auditioning the finger puppets

Dialing the rotary phone

Beating around the bush

Brushing the beaver

Digging a trench

Roughing up the suspect

Badgering the witness

Having a dry quilty (masturbating under the covers)

Spread Eagle

Spread the news: This position allows for maximum genital access! Lie on your back with your butt against a wall. Spread your legs, bend your knees, and rest the soles of your feet on the wall. From here, reach down to stimulate the vulva or clitoris.

Elle's Big Girl Move

When the hips are elevated with pillows underneath, the entire genital region opens up and the flesh on the stomach shifts back toward the chest and out of the way of the vulva. For those with an ample midsection, this can provide easier access, especially when your legs are spread and your knees are bent upwards.

    If you have a large tush, lying on your back can be uncomfortable, as it can place pressure on the lumbar spine. Adding enough pillows under your knees (if you're lying flat, or under your hips if you're spread eagle) until your back feels comfortable takes pressure of the spine. Pillows are a recipe for easy-access self-love, as they will raise your hips and bring your genitals closer to your hands.

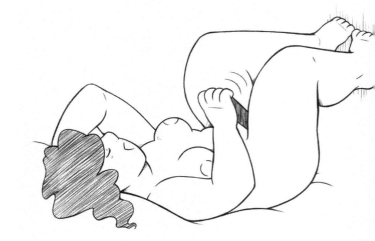

Want to use a toy while reclining and don't want to use your hands? Get comfy on your back, place a fluffy pillow between your knees, and wrap your legs around it tightly. Using lube, insert the dildo or vibrator of your choice so that the pillow is against the base of the toy. Lie back and thrust your body against the toy using the legs and pillow for leverage. The pillow-between-your-legs thrust motion works well on your stomach, too.

Side Saddle

This is a favorite solo sex position for many curvy gals because of its comfort and easy access for self-stimulation either by hand or with a vibrator. Lie on your side with your top leg bent and foot placed on the bed in front of your bottom leg for stability. In this position, there's room for the arm to reach down in front of you to stimulate the clit manually or with a vibrator, or even penetrate with a dildo.

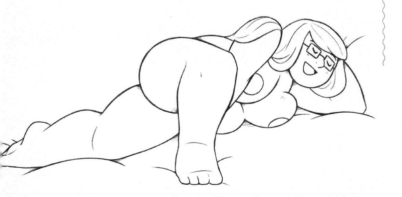

"My mother put her entire life on hold because of her weight. She refused to travel, date, or go on outings with friends until 'after she got thin.' Because her self-worth was so tied up in her appearance she died having missed countless opportunities. Growing up I became a casualty of my mom's insecurities and it had lasting effects on my self-image. Most days it's a challenge to accept my body the way it is and sometimes I have to really push myself to do things out of my comfort zone.

When I'm struggling I try to focus on this: Throughout my 44 years I've been various sizes ranging from medically underweight to morbidly obese. Reflecting back on all my positive life experiences, I recall how happy I was at that moment, not my appearance or size. Memories are just as wonderful whether I make them when I'm thin, fat, or somewhere in between. Remembering this helps me embrace whatever size I happen to be in the present and not let it stop me from living my life to its fullest."

Sunny Megatron, sex educator, star of Showtime's *Sex with Sunny Megatron*

Got Your Back

Lie on your back with your legs together and flat on the bed. Reach forward to stimulate your clitoris, vulva, or vagina. If your tummy is in the way, lift it and place your arms underneath so you can more easily reach your genitals.

"For 34 years I couldn't accept my body as it always was—fat. I also couldn't accept my sexuality. Too many years of shame built up into a lot of anxiety and frankly anger. One day someone made me see myself through another set of loving eyes. I only wish I'd been more forgiving of myself long ago. Now, I can accept and celebrate what I am, a beautiful and sexual being. I live freely, having sex with men and women who adore my soft body as it is. I don't need to lose five pounds or wear lingerie or lipstick if I don't want to in order to have sex."

Erin Nelson

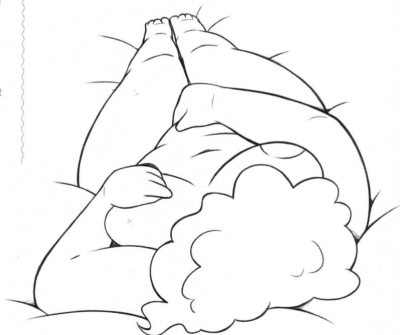

The Belly Dancer

Masturbating while lying on your belly can be very pleasurable but a little tough if you have a larger tummy. Again, pillows come to the rescue. To get into position, kneel on the bed, grab a fluffy pillow or two, and place it between your breasts and your stomach as you lie down. The pillow will cushion your stomach and elevate your torso enough to create a valley between it and your pelvis, allowing room for your hands or a wand vibrator.

Guided Masturbation and Imagery

There are lots of places on the Web to get information on masturbation. One of my favorites is Betty Dodson and Carlin Ross's website www.dodsonandross.com, which has a wonderful series of video clips called *Bodysex Workshops*. These clips not only teach women how to feel good about their sexuality, but also show *real* women (not actresses) with all different body types "taking care of business." Another validating website is www.ifeelmyself.com, a tasteful and artistic website that features women from all over the world masturbating to orgasm. It's liberating to watch women of all shapes, sizes, colors, and backgrounds enjoying themselves.

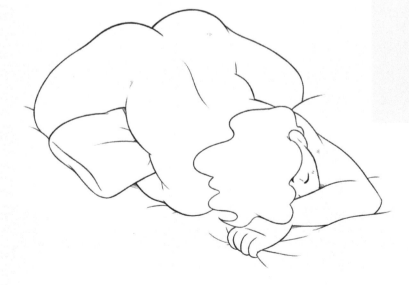

Sit / Stay

Who says you need to lie down to get off? Sitting up allows you to spread your legs as wide as you like, enabling you to reach your genitals more easily. One option is to grab a comfy chair and set the front of it about a foot from a wall. Have a seat, spread your legs, and rest your feet on the wall in front of you for leverage. You can do the same with any stable surface like a desk, a kitchen counter, or even the dashboard of your car (as long as you're not driving it!). Experiment with stretching one leg to the side, or resting a foot on the seat of the chair. If your tummy poses a challenge, select a chair that lets you recline a bit. Softening the angle between the torso and the pelvis will provide a more permissive entry for your hands. Letting the underneath of your tummy rest on your arms as you reach downward also works well, or try it with a wand vibrator.

"I can't count the number of women I've talked with who assume that because their desire is responsive, rather than spontaneous, they have 'low desire'; that their ability to enjoy sex with their partner is meaningless if they don't also feel a persistent urge for it; in short, that they are broken, because their desire isn't what it's 'supposed' to be. What these women need is not medical treatment, but a thoughtful exploration of what creates desire between them and their partners. This is likely to include confidence in their bodies, feeling accepted, and explicitly erotic stimulation. Feeling judged or broken for their sexuality is exactly what they don't need—and what will make their desire for sex genuinely shut down."

Emily Nagoski, Ph.D., from her best-selling book,
Come As You Are: The Surprising New Science
that will Transform Your Sex Life

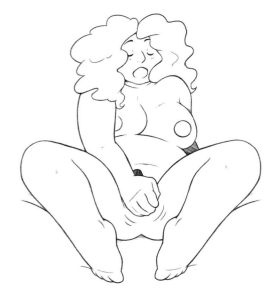

Singing in the Shower

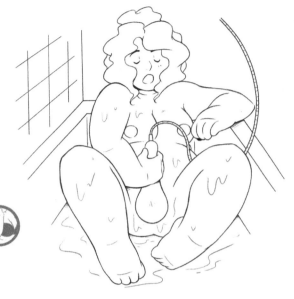

Get a little dirty while you're getting clean! The shower is a great place for solo sex. If you're using your fingers, grab a *tiny* bit of silicone lube or coconut oil—*not* soap—to make your fingers glide. Just be careful when you're done, as the tub may be slippery from whatever you're using. A handheld showerhead can be a curvy orgasm-seeker's best friend. While standing, aim the stream of water toward your clitoris, vulva, or anus. Experiment with different settings, from a light trickle to a throbbing pulse to find the perfect pressure for your pussy. In the mood for a bath? Hold the showerhead under the water, and when orgasmic nirvana hits, just tell your roommate you were singing in the shower.

Elle's Big Girl Move

Bath time fun is soothing and sexy. But let's face it: not everyone's tub or shower is built the same way—and for that matter, neither are we! I suggest purchasing some suction-cup handlebars and foot pedestals, which you can find easily online or from a medical supply store. Not only are these items great help for getting in and out of a tub, but they are moveable, so you can place them anywhere, for any reason. Showering with your partner? Have him pound away while you hold on tight to a handle, or bend your knee and place your foot on a suction cup foot pedestal. Feeling like going solo? Use that same foot pedestal to open up your nether regions so the water stream hits more surface area. When you're done, keep your foot steady on the pedestal while you shave your legs!

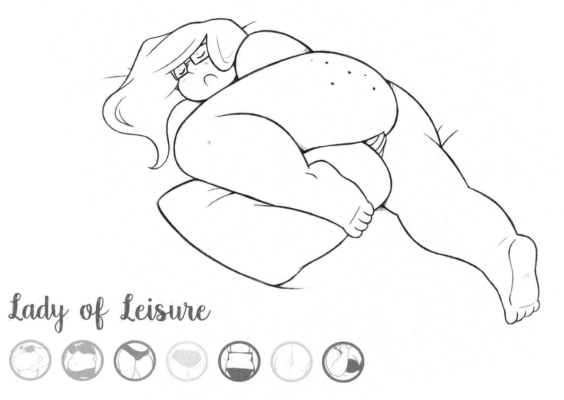

Lady of Leisure

Get comfortable in this luxurious self-love pose! Lie on one side with your top leg bent and your knee pressed as close to your chest as is comfortable. (If you like, you can place a pillow or two under the bent leg for support.) From here, your top arm can go south and stimulate your clitoris, vulva, or anus with a hand or a toy.

"The difference between a self-induced orgasm and an orgasm given by a man is like comparing a rainy day and a rainstorm. Rain was a sure thing; you knew exactly what you were going to get: a clean and crisp, both sweet and refreshing experience. But rainstorms were unpredictable; they were riddled with surprises, messy and wet; they were something you had no control over."

Madeline Sheehan

Solo Doggy

Be a lone wolf and get down in doggy style! Assume the position: on all fours, with the knees spread wide. To stimulate yourself, use a hand, an external vibrator, a dildo, rabbit vibe, or butt plug. If this is an uncomfortable position to stay in for a long time, utilize some of doggy variations shown in Chapter 7, or rest your torso on some fluffy pillows and extend your arms underneath you to get the job done.

Elle's Big Girl Move

Interested in a little solo anal stimulation, but your reach is limited by some body parts? Let the fetish world lend a hand! Fetish stores and websites carry a toy called an anal hook (don't worry, it's not sharp!). Usually used for BDSM play, this long and strong stainless-steel hook has a steel ball or balls connected to the end of the curve of the hook, and the long handle of the toy usually has a steel ring attached to the other end. Using that ring as your handle, you now have the extra length needed to reach and enter your well-lubed anus with the ball on the other end. Get into any position you like for solo play with the anal hook; doggy style, on your back, on your side—whatever feels comfortable. Just make certain you have lube by your side so you can reapply as needed.

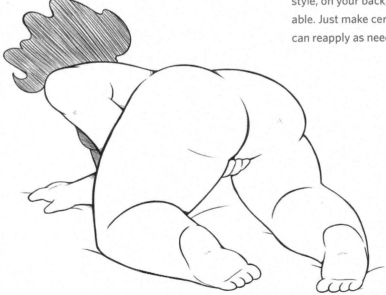

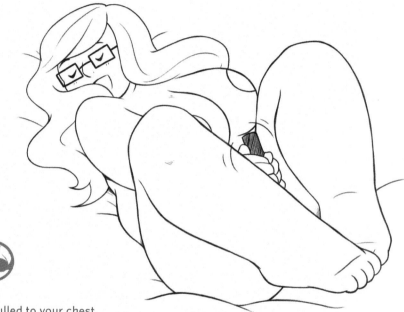

The Scarab

Lie on your back with your knees pulled to your chest. Spread your legs just enough to get your dominant arm between them to stimulate the clitoris, vulva, or anus with your fingers or a toy. It's no surprise that lot of curvy gals find this to be a preferred way to have solo sex. By bending, spreading, and pulling back your legs, your genitals are wide open and exposed, making it easier to rub your clit, stroke your labia, and stick your fingers in your vagina or ass.

Elle's Big Girl Move

Remember the wand vibrator I talked about in Chapter 2? The lengthy handle of a wand is a perfect match with any of these solo positions. If you find that some positions require some reach, the wand's length coupled with the power of something like the Original Magic Wand, or the length and angle of the Tantus Rumble, could mean the difference between being frustrated and being satisfied.

Flowering Lotus

If you're flexible and you know it, the Flowering Lotus is a fun, advanced position to experiment with. Sitting upright on your knees, spread your legs apart as wide as is comfortable. Leaning backward, support yourself with one arm and use the other to arouse your clit with your fingers or a vibrator. This is also a wonderful position for using a rabbit vibe for internal and external stimulation. Experimenting with different angles in this position might lead you to discover new postures and sensations that you might never have uncovered.

"Learn to be comfortable in your own skin. I like to hold, rub, and explore my curves. I know what feels good to me, and I've grown to love parts of my body that I used to hate, like my thighs and belly! Now I'm able to caress and touch them in ways that make me feel sexy. Loving my body makes being naked with a partner less stressful, so I'm able to stay present and not get caught up in my head. The more I appreciate my curves, the sexier I feel!"

LaTerra McDaniels, board member and educator, Center for Positive Sexuality, Los Angeles

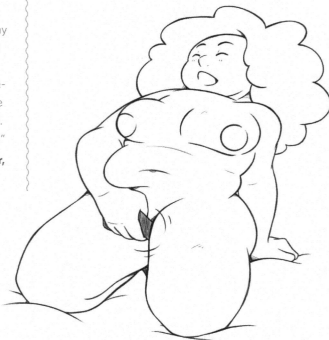

Chapter 5

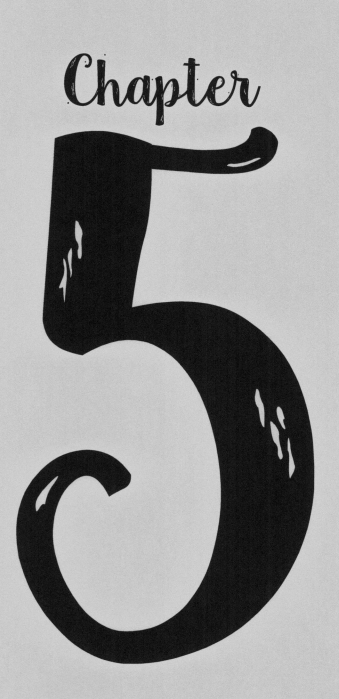

Learning to have sex from porn is like learning to drive from an action movie. Somebody is going to get hurt.

**Charlie Glickman, Ph.D.,
sex and relationship coach**

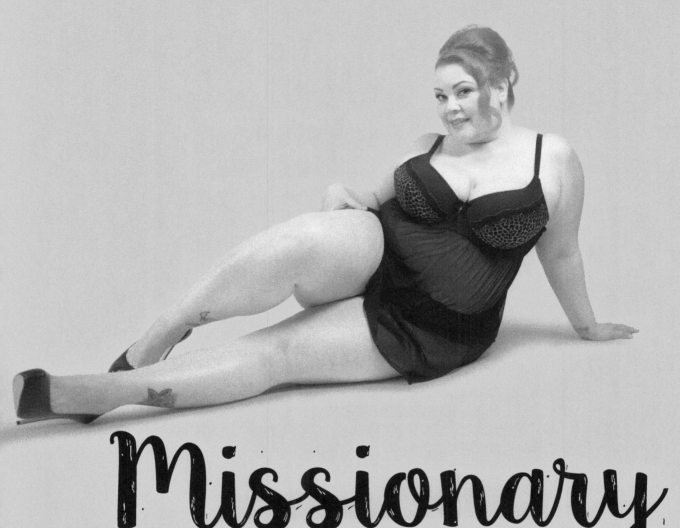

Missionary
TO THE MAX

It might surprise you to know that the missionary position is most women's favorite position.

Missionary may seem boring at first glance, but it is also one of the most versatile positions for a curvy girl. There are endless ways to modify it and take it to new levels.

There are a slew of reasons why missionary (or "mish") is a top pick. Some folks feel that being eye-to-eye with their lover makes for some deliciously intense intimacy. To others, the sultry, sensual feeling of another person's skin pressed against their own is a huge turn on. Then, there are people for whom the feeling of being under their lover—overtaken, enveloped, or enfolded in their arms—makes them weak in the knees.

Even so, missionary has its detractors. Some think of missionary as boring or "vanilla." For them, missionary means quick, serviceable sex, probably planned on a weeknight, where the woman just lies on her back and the man does all the work. To them I say, "Use your imagination!"

In truth, missionary is the queen of all sex positions. First of all, in this position, gravity works in your favor in any variation. When you lay back, all of your softer and curvier parts do, too. There's less to get in the way because gravity wants it to hang back. Also, because missionary is easily customizable, it has the potential for making plus-size sex more creative and exciting. As a bigger woman myself, I used to be a little worried about missionary. *What if my stomach gets in the way? What if my thighs are too big for him to get between?* Well, I've figured it out. If you are having the same feelings, not to worry—I'm here to make your frets and fears vanish.

Traditional Missionary

Sometimes called male dominant or male superior, traditional (heterosexual) missionary is generally any position where the man is on top of (or above) the woman. The classic way to achieve this is for the receiver to lie flat on her back with her legs spread in a V. The giver kneels between the receiver's thighs, and while resting his bodyweight on his hands/arms, he lowers himself over the receiver, aligning his pelvis with hers. The giver can either stay above, or gently rest on top of the receiver.

Sounds simple, right? It can be. But what if your tummy covers your mons and the top of your vulva? Or maybe it's throwing the alignment off? This could make clit stimulation a challenge, and a lot of woman need clitoral stimulation to come. In traditional missionary, clit stimulation can be tricky, but it can be achieved by placing a bullet vibe or other small, strong vibrator on your clit in between you and your partner. Alternately, whoever has a free hand—usually the receiver in this position—can simply place that hand in between both of you and rub while the other partner thrusts.

For those of us with ample bellies, we might find it easier to use a vibrator with a long handle, such as a wand (see page 33). When getting into position, use one of your hands to lift your tummy up and away from your mons and vulva. With the other hand, locate the controls on the wand and make certain your fingers are ready to control the speed, intensity, and/or patterns. Place the head of the wand on or near your clit and (if you like) release your tummy to fall where it may, which may help hold the wand in place. Voilà! Clit vibration is literally at your fingertips!

Elle's Big Girl Move

In general, I've found that giver-dominant positions, such as missionary, where the giver is lighter (or has a different weight distribution) than the receiver, can be more successful. If the weight balance makes this position difficult for you or your partner to enjoy, try a few variations but don't suffer through it. You might find that a female-superior, side-by-side, or doggie-style position is your reliable, magic, go-to pose. The good news is there are lots to choose from, so don't get discouraged!

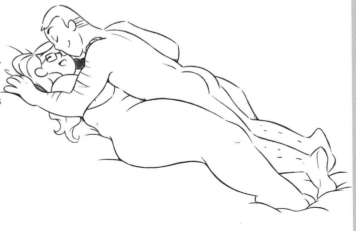

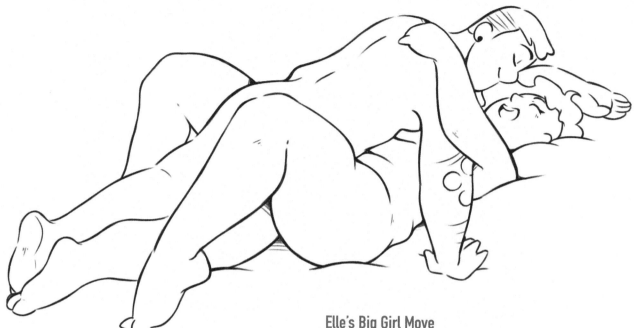

The Swan

Starting in the traditional missionary position, with the giver lying on top and between your legs, raise and bend your knees so your feet are flat on the bed and knees are pointing upward astride his hips.

Elle's Big Girl Move

When getting into position, women with larger stomachs might have to pull their tummy back to make room for their partner. There is no shame in doing this—it's an efficiency move, like tying back your hair to give a blow job or lifting your boob for him to suck. When it comes to clit stimulation in the Swan, the spirit of resourcefulness will be your saving grace. When moving your stomach away from the mons, take that opportunity to move your hand down to your clit. When the action begins, you already have a head start on arousal using your fingers or a bullet vibe.

Hugging the Curves

This position gives the receiver, a lot of control. Beginning in traditional missionary, wrap your legs around the giver; your feet may even touch or could rest against his lower back. This position takes advantage of the receiver's natural impulse to wrap their legs around his hips or waist to help him penetrate as deeply as he can. For even more command over depth, with your legs wrapped around his butt, you can use your heels for leverage and push him in even deeper, should you choose.

Elle's Big Girl Move

There are many possible varieties of Hugging the Curves. For gals with larger butts, leaning the back up on the headboard a bit and/or elevating the torso with pillows slightly will allow the giver to thrust while using his hands to stabilize himself against the wall or headboard. It's possible this adjustment can bring more friction to the receiver's clit (and the giver's if she has one) as well as make this move easier on the receiver's back.

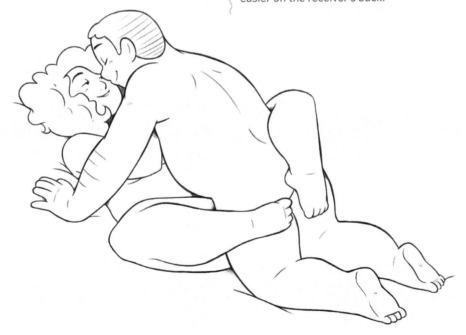

Fifth Position

You might notice this pose resembles fifth position in ballet, but I'm not going to be as strict as your childhood dance instructor. This modified missionary position uses a slight leg adjustment. The receiver keeps her knees horizontal on the bed while splaying her legs out to a V-shape position and then bringing her feet inward as if to touch. Like in missionary, the giver lies on top and between the receiver's legs, supporting himself with his arms. You can achieve clitoral stimulation with your hand, your partner's hand, or a small-but-powerful vibrator.

Elle's Big Girl Move

The key word here is comfort. Try this position by yourself first to see if it's a comfortable way to lie without the weight of someone on top of you. To mimic the pressure of another body, press down on the inside of each knee with your hands. If you feel muscle strain in your inner thighs, do daily stretches to make it more comfortable. Loosen up the inner thighs by mimicking the position while lying or sitting, or sit with legs crossed or feet together—press the knees down as long as it's comfortable and try to go further each time. This exercise will make you more limber, and the position more comfortable over time.

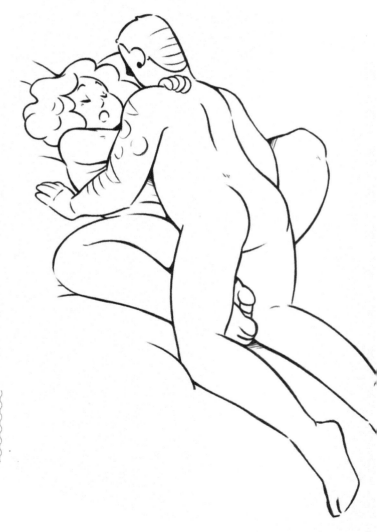

The Seashell

For the Seashell, start in the Swan position with your partner in between your bent legs. Then lift your legs—or have your partner lift them—to place them on his shoulders as far as comfortably possible. As a big girl myself, I love this tried-and-true position. If you have a larger stomach, manually pull back your tummy when getting into the Seashell. That way, as the giver begins to enter you, your thighs are in place holding the flesh away from the action for easier entry. If you like deeper penetration, the Seashell is right up your alley. Because your hips are lifted higher, your partner will find he has more room to move and will be able to position his body to get at just the right angle for his pleasure—and yours. For some, the Seashell can also be fantastic for G-spot stimulation, especially if your lover has a curve to his penis or is using a dildo with a curve. The angle of this position doesn't lend itself too well to clitoral stimulation. However, because the vulva is more exposed in the Seashell, the clit is more easily accessible for either of you to massage manually or use a bullet vibe or strong vibrating wand on, as he rides you into orgasmic nirvana. Some of us with sore shoulders or a stiff neck may want to put pillows under your head and shoulders. For those of us who don't bend as easily as we used to, this could be a position to work toward. As always, listen to your body and don't suffer through sex in an uncomfortable position.

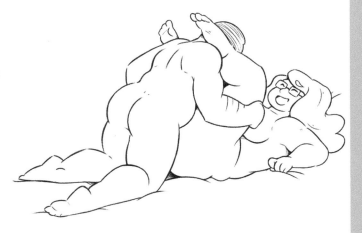

Elle's Big Girl Move

This is another position where—let's face it—you're just going to have to move your folds. There, I said it. The Seashell position is a lover of lift. By placing pillows or a Liberator Wedge under your butt and elevating your hips at a higher angle, you're practically presenting your vulva to your partner on a platter. Making this position convenient and easy-to-access for him gives him more choices. He can kneel and enter you, hold on to your feet at his shoulders (while sucking on a toe), or straighten out his legs like he would if he were doing push-ups, support his weight with his arms and press his hips into yours. The world is your oyster with the Seashell!

The Side Sash

Start in the Seashell position, with the receiver's knees bent and thighs against her chest. The receiver then brings her legs together and places them to one side of his head, resting on his shoulder (she can cross her ankles if that's more comfortable). He kneels in front, holding on to her crossed ankles (or not) and supporting himself with his other hand on the headboard, wall, or bed. He then lowers himself to an angle where his penis is aligned with her vulva and makes entry.

This is another terrific position for deep penetration, especially if you and your partner experiment using all the different angles this position can create with pillows, switching shoulders, or straightening out your knees. He probably won't be able to rouse the clit while working his hips and holding himself up, so again, you may need to lift your stomach and place your hand in position while holding a bullet vibe to your clit or rubbing it yourself.

Elle's Big Girl Move

Good news for foot fetishists! Your feet will be right next to his face, so if he has a thing for feet, he'll be in heaven! I love how high heels look (and so does my partner), but I loathe wearing them. However, when my legs are up in the air, I'm more than happy to don some sexy stilettos. I keep a gorgeous pair or two of heels in my closet for those times I want to titillate him.

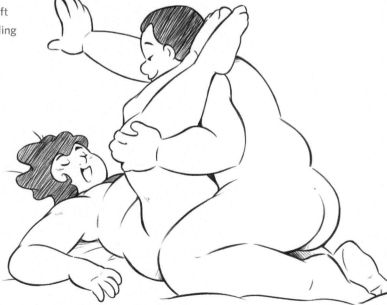

Threading the Needle

Your partner doesn't have to have a foot fetish to like this fun and deeply satisfying pose. It's easy to accomplish and a breeze to transition into from any woman-on-bottom position. To Thread the Needle, the receiver lies with her back flat against the bed and lifts her legs straight up. The giver kneels behind her and places her legs on each of his shoulders. He can either hold on to her knees, thighs, or hips while he thrusts, or he can use one hand to hold a leg and use the other hand to stimulate her clit. This is a wonderful position for her because both of you have at least one hand free for clit, nipple, and/or anal stimulation. Plus, he gets a lovely view of all the action.

Elle's Big Girl Move

Threading the Needle lends itself very well to placing a pillow under the hips. Make certain that the pillows are firm enough to elevate the hips approximately 6 inches (15.2 cm; lower or higher depending on comfort). The pillows tilt your hips high enough to let gravity work its magic and direct away from the genitals any flesh that might regularly be a challenge to move.

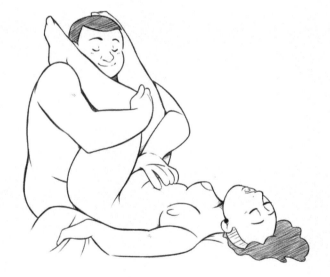

The Z

The giver kneels and sits back on his legs. Facing him, the receiver straddles his lap as she sits, then lies back with her butt and lower back supported by his thighs while she raises her legs in the air. The giver holds her legs, resting each one of her ankles on his shoulders, or holding them together in the air. The giver can move his hands to hold on to her thighs or hips, so he can control his thrusts into her by raising or lowering his body. Because the receiver's body is at a favorable angle, gravity will pull most extra flesh from her nether region giving everyone clear access to stimulate her clit.

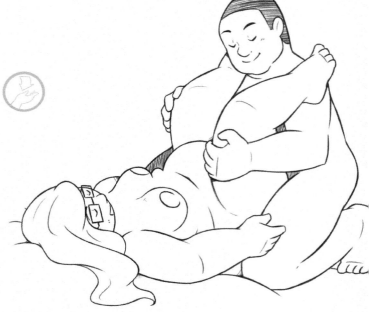

Elle's Big Girl Move

Another great variation to The Z is that instead of the receiver placing her ankles on his shoulders, she keeps her straight legs in the air, forming a *V*. The giver then uses his hands on her inner thighs to gently widen the *V* as he enters her. This is a terrific hack if those big, beautiful thighs are making this position a challenge, or if the giver likes to watch penetration—or his partner—during the throes of passion.

The Cup and Saucer

Start in the Z position, with the receiver's butt and lower torso on the giver's thighs; however, instead of the receiver placing her ankles on his shoulders, she bends her knees and places each leg on either side of the giver, with her feet flat on the bed. This position opens up her vulva more, giving him greater opportunity for entry. Again, the receiver's clit is readily exposed in this position, so either one of you can stimulate, rub, or tease it to delightful oblivion.

Elle's Big Girl Move

The giver has all of the control in this position, with the receiver prone and dependent on her partner to move her toward his penis. But this doesn't mean the receiver is passive and can't participate in all the fun. She can stimulate her own clit with her fingers, or take advantage of a prime opportunity to use one of those vibrators I mentioned in Chapter 2. In fact, because it gives you maximum length to work with, a wand vibrator like the Original Magic Wand or the Doxy massager is what I would recommend here. While your partner is thrusting, you can decide when and for how long you use the wand. What a feeling of power!

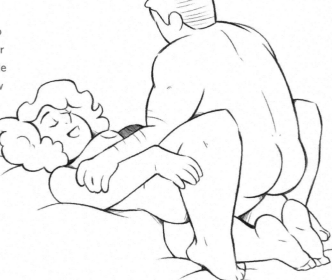

The Pogo Stick

Sitting back on his knees, the giver spreads his legs open enough to allow the receiver to sit in between. Facing the giver, the receiver fits herself in between the giver's legs, placing her legs over his thighs. The receiver then reclines with her back to the bed, and places one foot on his chest, leaving the other stretched out behind him.

Elle's Big Girl Move

If an aching lower back is a concern, placing a pillow or two underneath the receiver's butt, and maybe one under the shoulder blades, will help a lot. If pillows alone don't cut it, then try leaving the pillows in place and wrapping both legs around the giver's waist for more stability and control. In this position, the giver has the option of taking the receiver's hips in his hands and guiding the movement and the depth of penetration.

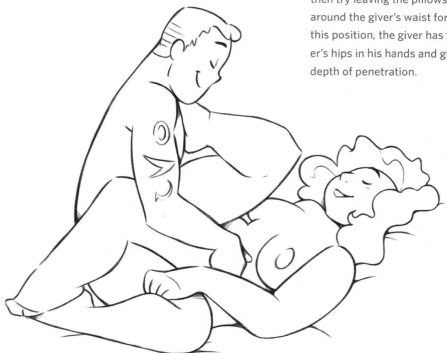

X Marks the Spot

Similar to the Side Sash, the receiver lies back on the bed, with her butt at the edge. She raises her legs and crosses them at the knees. The giver stands behind her and holds on to her legs while he thrusts. Depending on the height of the bed, X Marks the Spot can be a sensational way of varying missionary. This move requires minimal flesh adjustments, but the receiver has her hands free to move soft parts away from the action if needed.

Elle's Big Girl Move

Since there are varying heights of beds and people out there, use pillows to your advantage to raise the receiver's hips. Or if the bed is low to the ground, put them under the giver's knees so they can kneel comfortably. You also don't have to limit yourself to the bed—any stable and strong elevated surface will do, like a dining room table, the stairs, a desk… Let your imagination run wild!

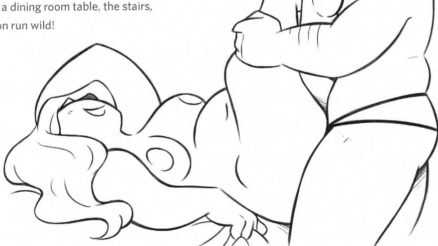

The Butterfly

If the receiver is flexible, this position is a fun one for all involved! The receiver lies on her back, with each ankle as close to the side of her head as possible; she can use her hands or arms to keep them in place. The giver kneels, aligns himself, then lies atop her, supporting himself with his arms. This position opens up the receiver's genital area to the giver's penis or dildo vaginally or anally, and can provide the giver a feeling of total control.

Elle's Big Girl Move

For some light BDSM play, try some straps! Usually called a sex sling or a slingshot, this webbed nylon strap comes with a wide padded panel in the middle and padded ankle cuffs on each end (see page 39). The padded panel goes across the back of the receiver's shoulders, while the ankles are secured in the ankle cuffs. The straps at the cuffs are adjustable, so you can set the angle that is most comfortable for you. Because the straps hold the ankles in place, this leaves the receiver's hands free to roam— perhaps to stimulate the clit, hold the tummy, or play with the nipples.

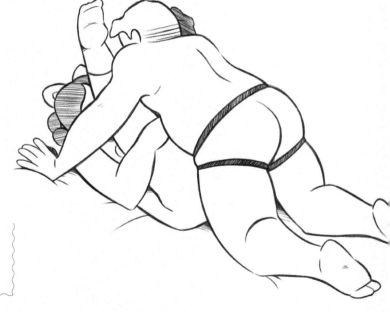

The Slingshot

The receiver lies on her back with one leg straight and the other leg bent with her foot flat on the bed. The giver kneels, straddling the thigh that's flat on the bed and holding on to the bent knee for leverage while he enters. For larger tummies, the receiver may find it useful to pull her belly back toward her or use a pillow under her hips so the tummy moves in the opposite direction.

Elle's Big Girl Move

Should the giver wish, he can manipulate the receiver's bent knee closer to her torso, or off to the side to get better access for penetration, or for different sensations for both of you. If it strikes his fancy, the giver might feel the urge to place the receiver's bent knee on his chest while grasping the receiver's hips for passionate propulsion here and there, for even for more control. In addition, feel free to try a pillow or two to switch the angle for even more variation. Any way you sling it, this is a fun position you'll want to revisit again and again.

Criss/Cross

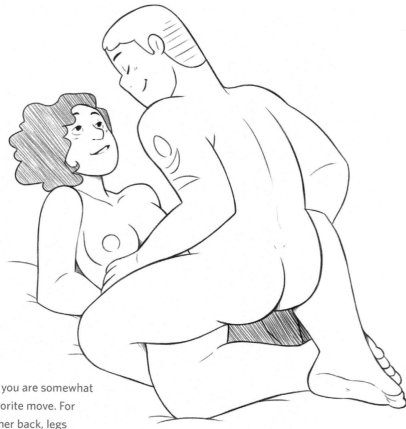

If you like deeper penetration and both of you are somewhat limber, Criss/Cross could be your new favorite move. For this advanced position, the receiver is on her back, legs flat but knees bent to the side and widely parted, and feet crossed at the ankles. Facing the receiver, the giver straddles her hips, aligns his twig and berries, wedges his ankles under her thighs, and presses his pelvis against hers when entering. Both of your hips are in close proximity in this position, so use it to your advantage. The receiver can grind against the giver's pelvis when he thrusts, which makes clitoral stimulation more likely. If tummies are being stubborn, the receiver can lift hers up for the duration or just after he enters. Either way, if you can do it, this intimate move will leave you breathless with passion.

Elle's Big Girl Move

If you are able to get into Criss/Cross easily, the receiver might want to elevate her torso with a pillow a bit for comfort. Don't be discouraged if this position feels more challenging than others, or if the important parts don't align well. Not every one of these positions is going to work for you, and that is perfectly fine. Sex is supposed to be fun, not stressful, so if this one isn't for you, move on to the next.

Stand and Deliver

The receiver sits with her butt at the edge of the bed and her feet touch or point toward the floor. She then lies back on the bed and brings her knees to her chest as close as is comfortably possible. The giver stands in front of her, grasps her legs for leverage, and enters.

Elle's Big Girl Move

Don't fret if at first you don't line up perfectly; that's what pillows are for! Strategically placed under the receiver's hips, a pillow can raise the vulva to a more conducive angle for entry. But the giver can help out, too. The giver can use one arm to gently hold the receiver's knees close to her chest, and use his other hand to raise the receiver's hips enough to enter comfortably *and* get a nice grasp of ass! This is also a terrific angle for anal penetration. Just make certain you go slow and use lube.

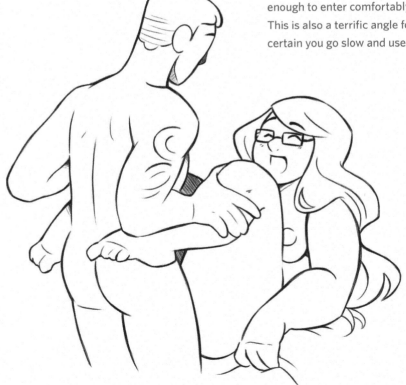

The Lumberjack

This position is great for deeper penetration and for the giver to take control. The receiver sits with her bum at the edge of the bed, with her feet dangling off the side. She then lies back and spreads her legs to allow the giver to get in between. The receiver then wraps her legs around the giver's waist. The giver lifts and bends one knee, resting his foot on the bed for leverage, and enters.

By placing his foot on the bed and astride the receiver, the giver is better able to control his thrusts and the receiver's legs, making The Lumberjack perfect for experimenting with dominant/submissive role play.

Elle's Big Girl Move

Get your anthropomorphic kink on and really role-play this sucker! Imagine that the giver is the lumberjack and the receiver is the tree. Each thrust is another attempt at felling the tree. Or, if you're looking for something a little lighter, a lumberjack and the seductive woodland nymph meet in the cooling shade of the forest to consummate their forbidden lust. You can take turns playing the lumberjack, and afterward, share a knowing glance and giggle over breakfast with friends. Beard, plaid flannel shirt, and woodland setting are optional.

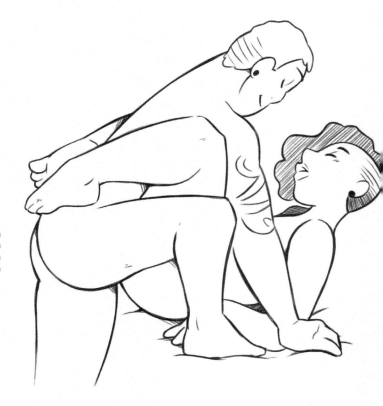

The Tree Hugger

Besides its name, the Tree Hugger has nothing to do with the great outdoors, but it is similar to the Lumberjack (page 82). The receiver sits with her butt at the edge of the bed and her feet dangling over the side. Lying back, she spreads her legs to allow the giver to get in between. The giver then bends to rest on top of her as the receiver wraps her legs around the waist or back of the giver. Tree hugging ensues. Now you have a way to celebrate mother nature.

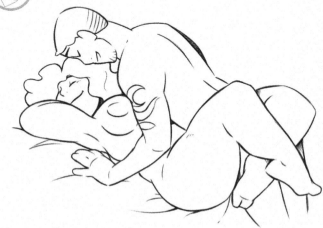

Your Vagina Is Not Silly Putty

Vaginal tissue does not stretch out with use, no matter how much you use it or how large the penis or toy is that it's used with. For comparison, think of your mouth and how it is stretched and manipulated every day, yet it always retains its shape—the same goes for your vagina. But like any muscle, the PC muscles that surround the vaginal canal can get weaker with age and after giving birth. Doing Kegel exercises regularly can help keep the PC muscles from losing their grip and might make your vagina *feel* tighter around a penis if clenched during sex.

Not certain how Kegel exercises work? You know how you clench to stop the flow of pee? That's a Kegel exercise. And, like just about everything else, there's an app for that. Check out the Emily Morse Kegel Camp app to keep those PC muscles fit!

The Love Letter

The receiver sits on the bed and crosses her legs. Then, keeping them in place, she lies back on the bed, bringing her crossed legs to her chest. The giver kneels in front of her and enters, lowering himself down on top of her and pinning her crossed legs to her torso. The crossed legs being pinned by the weight of the giver not only raises the hips a bit to meet the giver's cock or dildo, but it also opens up the thighs for easier access. You might find that a pillow under the hips of the receiver makes this position even more enjoyable.

Elle's Big Girl Move

This is an outstanding position for eye-gazing, tantric synchronized breathing, and mindful awareness of your partner's sexual responses. Because the giver is basically enveloping the entirety of the receiver's body with his own, this position can be very intimate as well as sexy. If the receiver wants that feeling of being overtaken in an all-encompassing bear hug, she can pull her arms into her chest and ask the giver to bring his arms in closer around her. If bellies get in the way, the receiver can try pulling back her stomach before the giver gets into place.

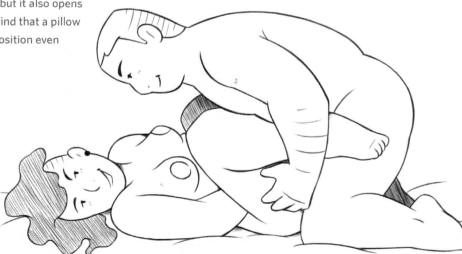

The Ohm

This delicious advanced position delivers deep penetration while playing with two different angles. The receiver begins by lying on her back and raising her legs in the air at a 90-degree angle. The giver sidles up to kneel right behind her, holding her legs close to his chest and lining up his pelvis with her vulva as he enters. After the giver has been in this position for a while, he moves the receiver's legs all the way to one side, yet the receiver's torso should stay turned upward toward the giver. The receiver should squeeze the PC muscles of her vagina during the position change to avoid the possibility of the giver slipping out. Whew! I'm getting a little warm just describing it!

Elle's Big Girl Move

This is my favorite position because of all the ways it can be customized. For instance, if you both have a big belly, you'll be happy to know that this position is for you! Because the giver is entering from behind, the receiver barely has to move her tummy away from the action, unless it is to make her more comfortable or to readjust where her tummy and thighs meet. The giver can bend the receiver's legs toward her torso more if his belly is challenging. Also, if the receiver has a prodigious ass, the giver has his hands free to push butt cheeks away from each other, push the outside leg of the receiver up toward her chest to open up the area a bit more, or just enjoy the view and use one of his hands to play with her clit.

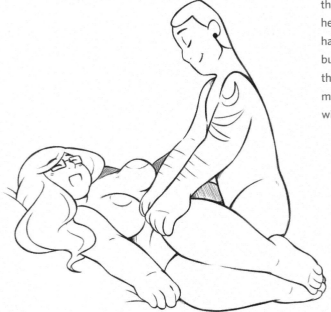

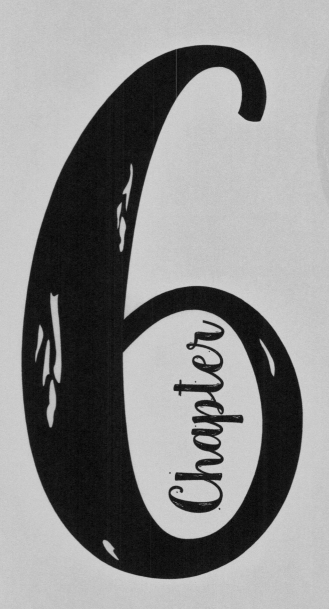

Chapter 6

No matter your size or shape, your body is built to receive pleasure. Take advantage of it. Far too much time has already been wasted by people waiting to change themselves before they'll enjoy themselves. I've done it, too. There's no dress size that will bring you confidence, because confidence is a state of mind, and it's the sexiest feature of all. So just start rocking what you've got. People will love it.

Stella Harris, sex educator and erotica author

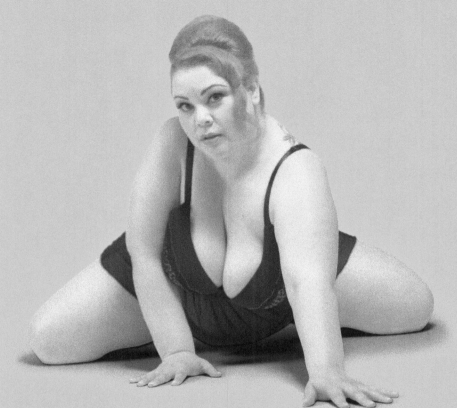

Be Gutsy and
GET ON TOP

If you're used to being the receiver on the bottom of a position, turn the tables and get in the driver's seat once in a while—it can be a nice change of pace!

If you like G-spot stimulation, you might find that receiver-on-top positions are more likely to make you sing, because at these angles, the G-spot is usually in the direct line of fire of the giver.

Still, others can find being on top uncomfortable for a variety of reasons. This is not uncommon, as no vagina is exactly alike, nor are our lovers' parts. Add to the equation our various ranges of flexibility, sizes, physical restrictions (like a bad back, for example), and you have myriad reasons why being on top might be challenging. But if you enjoy it, being on top can be empowering and sensual, and has the added benefit of letting your partner get a nice view of the action.

The Rocking Horse

In this advanced position, the giver kneels and sits back on his legs. With her back to him, the receiver straddles his thighs, bending her knees so that her legs are alongside his, and lowers herself down onto his penis. If she feels like it, she can lower her torso, too, using her forearms to help support her upper body. The giver can then use his hips to thrust inside her, and get even closer and deeper by bending his torso over her and holding on to her shoulders as he thrusts, thus "riding" her like a rocking horse. Placing firm pillows under the receiver's torso can help ease any back or neck pain that might occur.

Elle's Big Girl Move

To make room for larger tummies, he can spread his knees apart, or hold on to her thighs and sit up before thrusting. In the Rocking Horse, not only does the giver have easy access to her rear so he can spread her butt cheeks and stimulate her anus, but he can also rub her back or maneuver his hand under her to stimulate her clit. If he craves more control, he can hold on to her hips with one hand while holding himself up with the other.

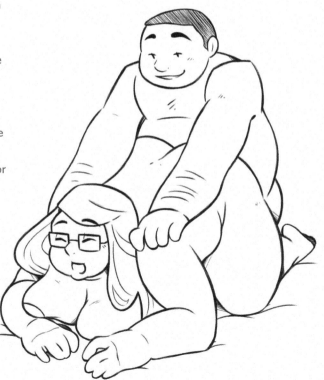

Yab Yum

This is a classic Tantra position that a lot of larger women are apprehensive about—but there's no need to be frightened; it's easier than you think and deliciously intimate. The giver sits cross-legged on the bed. The receiver sits in the giver's lap, facing him and with her legs wrapped around his waist or hips. Adjust yourselves as needed so that the giver can easily enter the receiver. Both of you thrusting slowly toward each other, or even rocking back and forth, builds a collaborative motion that can be incredibly erotic. This is a position that fosters closeness and intimacy, so embracing, kissing, and eye-gazing are highly encouraged.

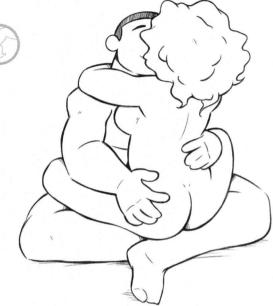

Vaginas Don't Gain Weight

Let me set the record straight. There is no truth to the trope that fat women have bigger vaginas. On average, regardless of body size or shape, the vagina in its unaroused state measures between 2.5 and 3.7 inches (6.4 and 9.4 cm) in length and varies along that span from approximately 1 to 2 inches (2.5 and 5 cm) in diameter. Every woman's vagina swells and engorges with blood when aroused. This elongates the vaginal canal and, in the process, causes the cervix and uterus to pull back, making room for a penis or toy to enter. This phenomenon—called vaginal tenting—can double the length of a woman's vaginal canal during arousal. It's also important to note that a woman's vaginal canal and cervix can fluctuate in size during the month depending on where she is in her cycle or pregnancy. This process is the same for all vaginas. If the vagina is sufficiently aroused, relaxed, and lubricated, it should take a cock or dildo with ease and, hopefully, enjoyment. However, if a vagina is not aroused enough to produce adequate lubrication, or the vagina owner is anxious or not ready to be penetrated, it can give a penis the impression that it's tighter.

Yum Yab

Guess what this position is a variation of? Yup, you guessed it. The Yum Yab is just like the Yab Yum, except instead of crossing his legs, the giver keeps his legs out straight in from of him. The receiver then sits in between the giver's legs, with her thighs atop his. The receiver can extend her legs or wrap them around the giver's back or hips, and even assist him in his thrusts for deeper penetration.

Elle's Big Girl Move

Just like in the Yab Yum position, in Yum Yab, the giver can place his hands under or behind the receiver's butt to pull her closer for more skin-to-skin contact or to aid in penetration. However, if at least one of the giver's hands aren't being utilized, he can use it to stimulate the receiver's clit or anus, or stroke whatever erogenous zone is closest. For her part, the receiver can put at least one hand to work by stroking the giver's chest, or even just holding him closer. Intimacy is the hallmark of this position, so set that intention when you're in it and let your instinct show you how to move, where to fondle, and how to connect more deeply with your partner.

The Lap Dance

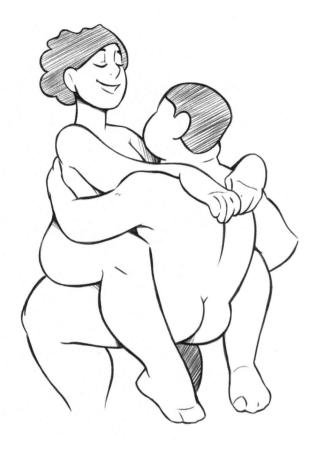

Grab a chair, because you're about to master a classic: the lap dance! With legs together, the giver sits in an armless chair. The receiver then straddles the giver's lap and lowers herself down onto a hard penis or strap-on while balancing herself by holding on to the giver's shoulders or the back of the chair. Grind away! The giver can spread and squeeze her butt cheeks, or go north and give "the girls" some attention. If your clit needs some action, either one of you can accommodate with a free hand.

Elle's Big Girl Move

Since this is a stripper's bread-and-butter move, why not take this opportunity to explore role-playing? Start by renting the campy *Striptease* or *Showgirls* to get into the mood. Think about how you might want to seduce your partner. Will you start with a grind and get them all worked up? Perhaps a little hand massage or oral appetizer before you really get into your lap dance? Do you want to strip, or keep your clothes on? Will you undress your partner first, or let them fidget in their clothes the whole time? It's completely up to you—but whatever you decide, I'm certain your partner will be very appreciative.

Reverse Lap Dance

Yep! Switch it around for a little variety mid-dance, and give your partner a nice view from the back. The giver sits, legs apart, in an armless chair. The receiver then stands between the giver's legs, facing away, and proceeds to lower herself down onto his hard penis or strap-on while keeping herself stabilized with her hands on the giver's knees, then twerk it, baby!

Elle's Big Girl Move

Feeling frisky on that road trip? Ever tried sex in a car? Both Lap Dance moves work great in your vehicle's backseat. Straddle the giver's lap facing forward or back, and grab the top of the seats for support. Rather than taking off your clothes, you can push panties to the side, lift up a shirt, or unzip pants and pull them down to the ankles. Clothes askew but still intact can give the encounter a feeling of an illicit rendezvous that could be discovered at any moment. So go ahead and steam up those windows before someone stumbles upon you!

Traditional Cowgirl

      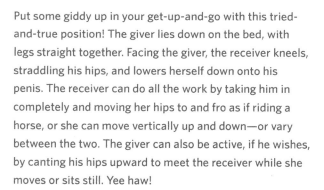

Put some giddy up in your get-up-and-go with this tried-and-true position! The giver lies down on the bed, with legs straight together. Facing the giver, the receiver kneels, straddling his hips, and lowers herself down onto his penis. The receiver can do all the work by taking him in completely and moving her hips to and fro as if riding a horse, or she can move vertically up and down—or vary between the two. The giver can also be active, if he wishes, by canting his hips upward to meet the receiver while she moves or sits still. Yee haw!

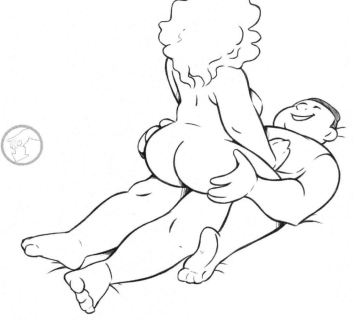

Elle's Big Girl Move

Imagine how it would feel to have your vulva lips lightly grazed by your partner's fingertips while you were super turned on. Good, right? Grazing your fingertips along your partner's balls gives him a similar feeling. If you know your partner likes to have his balls played with, try reaching one hand behind you to touch, feel, or skim them lightly with your fingers. For a lot of men, feeling this sensation while having sex can feel ah-mazing.

Horizontal Cowgirl

This position starts exactly like Traditional Cowgirl: The giver lies down on the bed, with legs straight together. Facing the giver, the receiver kneels, straddles his hips, and lowers herself down onto his penis. Now, instead of staying upright, the giver bends forward and rests her chest on his. In this position, they can both move in unison to a comfortable tempo, or either one can do the work. The receiver can push herself back on his penis, or her partner can pump away. Move your flesh on bigger tummies to accommodate, as necessary. Try lifting your tummy up as you lie down on your partner.

Elle's Big Girl Move

It doesn't get closer than this! Think about it: You are literally joined at the hips, chest-to-chest, face-to-face. The giver can wrap his arms around the receiver in a bear hug, lightly stroke her back, play with her hair, or kiss her; she can stroke his face, wrap her arms around his head, or hug him back. This is a position where you can really feel each other's heart rate and excitement. Try it while gazing into each other's eyes, or with your heads closer to each other in order to whisper sweet (and salacious) nothings to your partner.

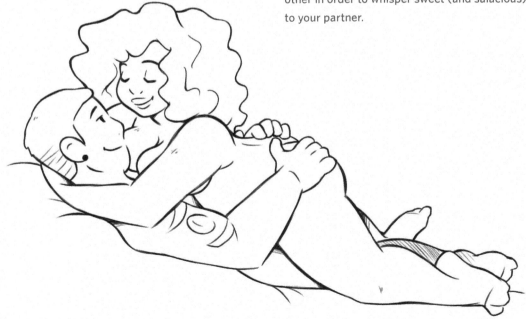

Reverse Cowgirl

The giver lies on his back, with legs straight. Facing away from him and kneeling, the receiver straddles his hips, and then lowers herself down onto his penis. Just like in Traditional Cowgirl, both partners can participate in the movement, it just depends on what you're up for! Receivers with lower-back pain might find this version of being on top more comfortable. If your lower back flares up, lean forward so your chest touches your partner's knees, if you have to, or you can use your knees for balance and leverage to bob your hips up and down on his cock. If thighs or butt cheeks get in the way, the giver is in a good position to lustfully clutch them and move flesh away from the vulva.

Elle's Big Girl Move

As long as you don't have a bad back, try varying your angle by leaning back and placing your hands on his chest or astride her torso for support. Another twist is to stay upright and squeeze your legs together. This will tighten up the muscles around your pelvic floor, which can sometimes supply the giver with a snugger feeling—also your hands are free to play with his balls or to stimulate your clit.

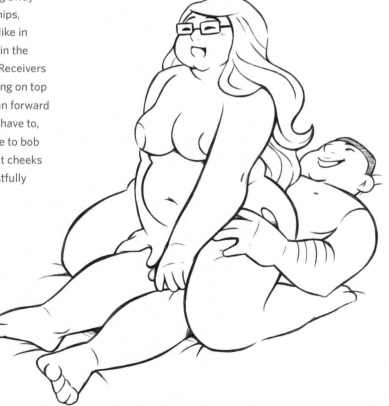

The Jockey

Pretend you're the jockey racing for the Triple Crown with this fun position. You might even want to take out your riding crop! The giver sits up on the bed, with his back against the wall or headboard and legs straight out in front of him. Facing away from him, the receiver straddles his hips and kneels with legs astride him, and then slides him into her. With your back to your partner, a bigger tummy won't be in the way and he gets to enjoy the view from behind. His hands are free to spread your butt cheeks, rub your neck and back, play with your breasts, or rub your clit using his fingers or a toy.

Elle's Big Girl Move

Just because you're not facing each other doesn't mean that this position can't be intimate. The Jockey is fun at a trot or a gallop. If you want something slow and sensual, lean back toward your mate as you sway your hips slowly to and fro. Want to pick up speed? Lean forward a bit, support yourself with your hands in front of you on his shins, or to your side, and twerk your tushy to your heart's delight.

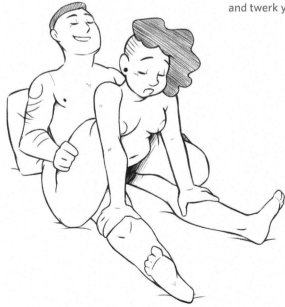

The Deck Chair

The giver sits on the edge of the bed, closes his legs together, sets his feet on the floor, and then lies back. Facing the giver, the receiver straddles his hips and bends her knees one at a time, placing them on the bed on either side of his hips. This is a terrific position if the receiver likes to be in control of thrusting and if she wants to experiment with body and hip angles for a variety of different sensations during penetration. Also, if the giver happens to be larger around his middle, this position allows the giver to be in a place where she can lovingly manipulate it to suit their needs so that his penis is more accessible.

No Longer a Drag

For any of the positions in this book, if your sweaty bodies are pushing and pulling your skin in uncomfortable or painful ways, slather some massage oil or even a bit of silicone lube on the vexing spots before you go chest to chest, hips to ass, or any other combination that has you tugging and rubbing each other's skin. It can be super-sensual to apply, and the slippery feeling as your bodies move against each other can be very erotic.

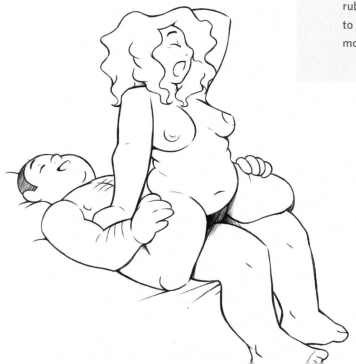

The Scenic Vista

For this advanced position, the giver sits up with legs out straight and pillows under his butt. The receiver straddles the giver's hips, allowing him to enter her, then straightens out her legs toward the giver's torso. For balance, the giver can hold on to the receiver's hips or hands. After the giver enters, he reclines completely, leaving the receiver to enjoy the extra penetrative depth achieved by having her legs out straight while on top. Should they choose, the giver may bend his knees to help support and balance the receiver. In the meantime, the giver gets a fantastic view to enjoy while thrusting or being thrust upon!

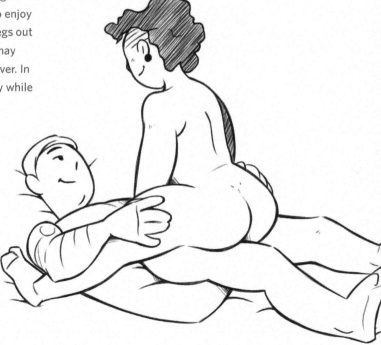

Chapter

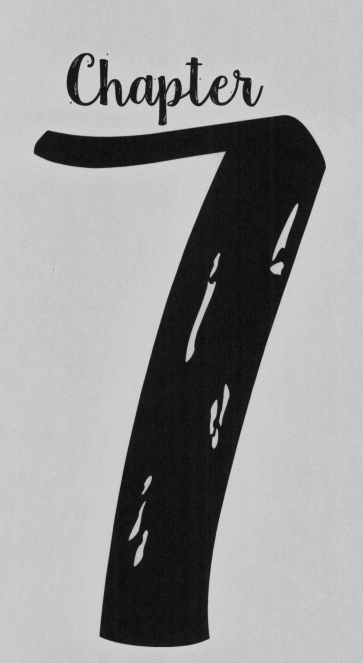

Loving your body exactly as it is
is an act of civil disobedience.

Catherine Deveny,
Australian writer, columnist, and activist

Coming from BEHIND

No book on sex positions would be complete without variations of getting banged from behind.

You may have heard that the classic position is called doggy style because it's the position that dogs (and many other mammals for that matter) mate in. Its versatility for manipulating body angles for people of size is unrivaled because not only is the receiver's tummy out of the way but the giver also has his hands free to spread cheeks and vulva, not to mention massage the clit. Doggy is also great for those who like the feeling of deeper vaginal and anal penetration, and if you are having anal sex, there simply isn't a more cooperative angle to do it in.

Traditional Doggy Style

The receiver is on her hands and knees, with legs spread wide. The giver kneels between the receiver's legs and enters from behind. The giver can hold on to the receiver's hips while thrusting, or use her hands to stimulate the receiver's breasts, clitoris, or anus. Likewise, the receiver can use a hand to self-stimulate or massage the giver.

Elle's Big Girl Move

If you like this position, invest in a Doggy Style Strap, which is a long stretch of nylon webbing with an oblong padded piece of fabric in the middle and handle loops on each end. The Doggy Style Strap is placed underneath the hips of the receiver, while the giver holds on to the reins. This accessory can provide the giver with more thrusting control and leverage, and gives the person being penetrated more stability and relieves the pressure on the back and wrists.

Top Dog

The receiver is on her hands and knees, with her legs together. From behind, the giver kneels while straddling the receiver's legs and enters. Because the receiver's legs are together, this position can make for more friction on a penis. The giver can also use his hands to squeeze her butt cheeks together as he's thrusting for a more snug sensation.

Elle's Big Girl Move

This position may be challenging for people who have bad knees or backs. To lighten the pressure on the receiver's back, have her rest her torso on pillows or a Liberator Wedge. Liberator also makes something called a "spanking bench," which is L-shaped and made out of the same sturdy industrial foam their other products are made from. The receiver would kneel on the lower part of the "L," cushioning the knees, and bend over the top part of the "L" while the giver enters from behind. Or you can get more creative and toddle over to the living room to bend over an ottoman or footstool.

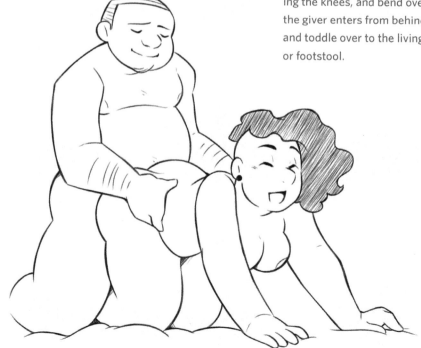

Wild Rover

The receiver is on her hands and knees, with legs spread wide. The giver kneels behind her on one knee, as if proposing. The knee that is down goes between the receiver's legs, and the opposite foot goes outside of the receiver's leg as he aligns his bits with hers and enters from behind.

Elle's Big Girl Move

Butt plugs are getting more popular among women nowadays and it's no surprise why. Because the wall between the anus and the vagina is so thin, some women report that the friction caused by having both orafices occupied at the same time (along with some gentle thrusting) is an enormously pleasurable and unique sensation. If this is something that's piqued your interest, the Wild Rover is a great position to try while using a butt plug. The giver can gently, slowly, and with a lot of lube, insert a plug of the receiver's choice into her anus. Remember to communicate with the giver when he's inserting the plug and go slowly—anal penetration should never hurt. Once the plug is in place and he has entered the receiver's vagina (with a penis or a dildo), the giver can use one of his free hands to stimulate her clit. If the butt plug and vaginal penetration is too intense the first time, try inserting the plug and not engaging in vaginal penetration, but stimulate the clit to orgasm or for as long as she's enjoying it. You might find that butt plugs make a gratifying addition to your sexual repertoire!

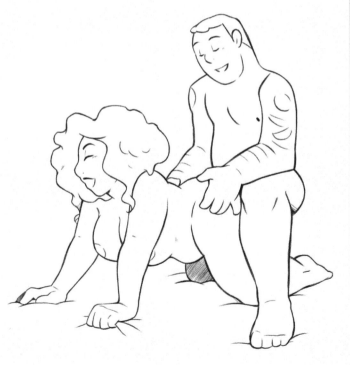

Downward Doggy

    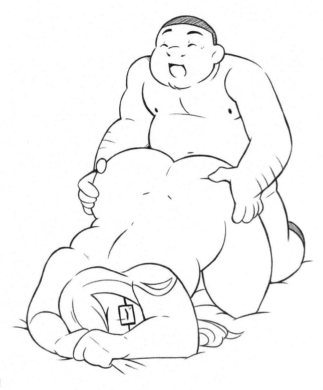

This advanced position might as well be called Deeper Downward Doggy for its ability to really enhance the feeling of deeper penetration. The receiver starts on hands and knees before straightening both the arms and legs so her butt is in the air and her body is in the shape of an inverted *V*, with hands and feet on the floor (like the Downward Dog pose in yoga). The giver stands behind the receiver's legs, aligns the genitals, and enters. In this position, gravity works in your favor to move tummies and butts that can sometimes impede performance. If Downward Doggy puts uncomfortable pressure on the receiver's wrists, she can bring her forearms to the floor.

Elle's Big Girl Move

They key to get the deep penetration experience is the level of each participant's hips. If the giver is on the shorter side, I recommend that the receiver rests on her forearms and knees instead of her hands and feet. Also, if the receiver enjoys a little anal stimulation, the giver can slap some lube on it and massage or (with permission) insert a finger while he's riding her.

Whoopie Pie

The receiver bends over the bed, keeping her legs together and supporting herself with her forearms. The giver stands behind the receiver, with one leg on either side of hers, and enters between the still-closed legs. The giver's hands are free to stimulate the nipples or clitoris, to do a little (consensual) slap and tickle, or to simply hold on tight while thrusting.

Elle's Big Girl Move

This is a pretty portable position, so why not venture outside the bedroom and take the Whoopie Pie elsewhere in the house? The receiver can just as easily bend over the arm of a sofa or the edge of a dining room table. The bathroom can also be exciting if the receiver bends over the counter so both participants can watch the action in the bathroom mirror.

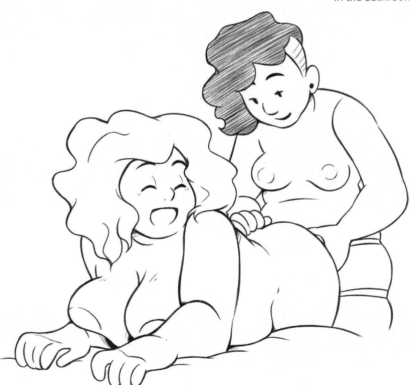

Tailgate

Sex educator and author of *The Anal Sex Position Guide*, Tristan Taormino coined the term "Tailgate" for this fun position. If you like to surf, you might already know that the term "tailgate" means to paddle out on your surfboard (or follow another surfer paddling out) to catch a wave. To configure a perfect Tailgate, the receiver lies flat on her stomach, with her legs slightly parted. The giver straddles her thighs and enters. Soon you'll be riding that wave together!

Elle's Big Girl Move

If the giver has a challenging time getting in, he's well situated to part the butt cheeks or thighs for more access. Alternately, pillows can be placed under the receiver's hips to tilt the backside up, which should make entry easier. Want more power in your push? Have the receiver place her arms at her sides so the giver can hold her hands and pull her toward him for extra leverage while thrusting.

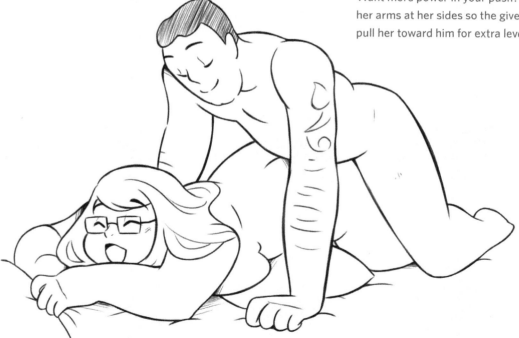

Dovetail

The receiver lies on her stomach, with pillows under her hips and legs spread. The giver kneels between the receiver's legs and enters from behind. The giver can remain upright, grab on to the receiver's hips, and thrust powerfully, or come forward to lie on his partner's back for a more sensual experience.

"Both men and women often ask, 'What's so great about anal sex?' The answer to that question involves both the physical experience and the emotional and psychological elements that come into play. Like sex in general, anal sex is a holistic experience that encompasses our bodies as well as our minds and our spirits. The opportunities for pleasure through anal play are diverse, and what makes one person moan with delight may leave another person uninspired. For most people, it is a combination of factors that make anal sex a satisfying activity."

Tristan Taormino, author of
The Anal Sex Position Guide

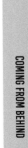

What, What, in the Butt?

It's worth noting that, unless otherwise specified, the positions in this book are intended for vaginal sex. However, many of the positions in this section are also great for anal sex (watch for the handy icon that identifies them). If you are new to backdoor action but excited to try, there are a few essential basics you should know:

- **Butt sex should *never* hurt.** Never. Never, ever, ever. If you're having anal sex and experiencing pain of any kind, at any time, STOP.

- **Use lubricant—lots of it.** The anus is not self-lubricating, so to make anal penetration comfortable you need lube—there are no two ways about it. In addition, the delicate skin in the anus is more susceptible to micro-tears than the skin in the vagina, and even more so without lube. This means that it's just that much easier to contract a sexually transmitted infection (STI)—and for my money, that's reason enough to use lube.

- **What kind of lube should you use?** Some people prefer to use a water-based lube (often in gel form), and others prefer the longer-lasting slip of silicone lube, but whatever you choose, have it within arm's reach and don't be shy about reapplying, especially when you're thinking butt sex could be on the menu for the evening.

- **No double dipping.** Never insert anything in the vagina immediately after it has been inserted in the butt to avoid introducing bacteria that could lead to infection. You can go from vagina to butt, but not butt to vagina. If you want to go from the "ass to the grass," wear a condom and switch to a fresh one in between.

- **Go *very* slowly.** This is especially important if you've never been penetrated anally before. Using some lube, allow your partner to start by massaging the outside of your anus (butthole) and the inside of your butt cheeks. When you're used to that, ask your partner to penetrate your anus slowly and incrementally with their finger bit by bit, over the course of a few sessions, so you (and your butt) can get used to the feeling.

- **Clitoral stimulation goes a long way when attempting anal.** In fact, some women cannot enjoy anal penetration without it.

- **Check in.** Both partners should talk with each other frequently about how it feels. Don't be distressed if it takes some time—done properly, it should.

Not everyone enjoys butt sex. If you try fingers, a dildo, or a cock, and you're not feeling it, there's nothing wrong with telling your partner that anal is not for you. After all, sex of any kind should be pleasurable, consensual, and fun, right?

Whether you're new to butt sex or whether you usually enjoy a finger in your tushy or have had enjoyable anal before, it's still possible to run into issues. If you're following all the steps (going slowly, using lube, wearing a condom) and it's still a challenge to gain entrance, there are a few reasons this might be happening. Check with your body:

- Are you tense? Are you uncomfortable physically, or not completely comfortable with your partner?

- Do you need to apply more lube?

- Is your position the best one for you and your partner's shapes and sizes?

If none of these questions lead you to the culprit, take heed: The doyenne of anal sex, Tristan Taormino, who is the author of several books on the subject, says, "Sometimes, the butt wants what the butt wants—and sometimes, that's not sex." In other words, don't force it, move on to something else, and try it again another time.

Wheelbarrow

Welcome the birds and the bees of spring by trotting out the good ol' Wheelbarrow. This advanced position requires the receiver to lay face forward on the bed with her legs dangling off the edge. The giver, standing behind her, maneuvers himself in between her legs and enters. Thrusting ensues and the giver uses his stamen to "pollinate" her flower. If the receiver's back hurts in this position, you can try placing pillows under her hips and giving her another pillow to clutch and rest her head on. If that doesn't relieve the issue, scrap this pose and try the Flying Wheelbarrow (page 121) instead.

Sphinx

Receiver starts by resting on her forearms and knees (see Whoopie Pie, page 107), with legs spread. The giver kneels outside or between the receiver's legs and enters from behind. The receiver has the option to remain active, using her arms to push her backside toward the giver, or to relax, resting her head on the bed (or floor or whatever surface she's on). This is another position that can be made more comfortable for the receiver by placing pillows under her chest to cushion her breasts and support her shoulders.

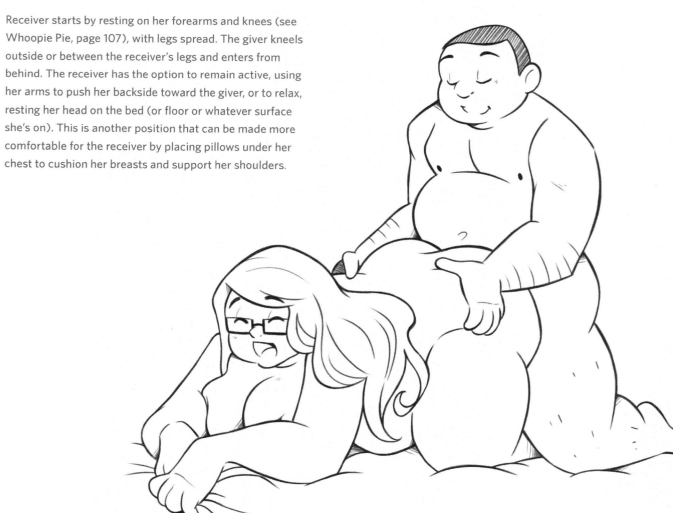

What a Pain

Sometimes, you can be really turned on, comfortable, and excited to try a rear-entry position, but when vaginally penetrated, it just hurts. Painful intercourse is called *dyspareunia* and can have a few different causes, from starting too fast to not enough lubrication to inflammation. Regardless, I recommend being examined by a health care professional to determine why you're experiencing pain during sex. If you only experience pain during rear-entry vaginal sex, you might be one of approximately 30 percent of women who have a tilted uterus. Sometimes referred to as a "retroverted" or "tipped" uterus, a tilted uterus means that instead of your uterus tilting towards the front of your body, it tilts toward the back (to some degree). It stands to reason that depending on many factors, like size and shape of the penis or dildo doing the penetrating and how vigorous the thrusts, women with a tilted uterus might experience pain or discomfort when doing it doggie style. The pain is usually caused by the penis or dildo poking the sensitive uterus, ovaries, or cervix (and can depend on where you are in your cycle). If any or all of these rear-entry positions seem to cause internal discomfort, take them out of your reportoire and check with your doctor—a retroverted uterus might be the culprit.

Reclining Sphinx

In this intermediate move, the receiver lies on her stomach on the bed and props her head and torso up with her forearms. She spreads her legs and pulls one knee into her chest. The giver straddles the straight leg on his knees, and then lies forward on top of her and enters. The giver can stay in that position, or use his arms to push up while thrusting.

Elle's Big Girl Move

The Reclining Sphinx is one of those positions that is good for both a vigorous tryst or something on the slower side. If you're feeling a little more intimate, the giver can rest his chest atop the receiver's back and wrap his arms around her. Instead of thrusting, the giver can employ a rocking motion with his hips and body, which can give the receiver a safe and secure feeling.

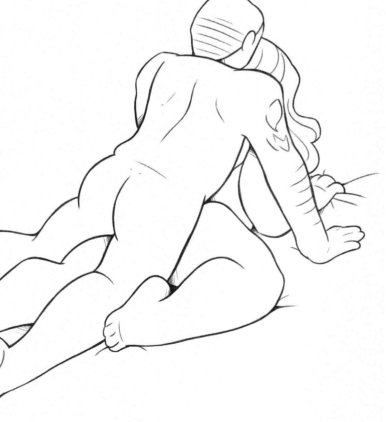

Go Deeper

Like its name implies, Go Deeper allows for just that: deep penetration. The receiver bends forward over the edge of the bed, with legs spread wide. The giver stands behind her with his feet between hers, and enters. This position creates plenty of opportunities to play with angles. The giver can use his dominant position to slightly turn his body outward to either side, allowing his penis to meet her vaginal walls at different angles. The giver should start slower in this case as certain angles might not be comfortable for the receiver.

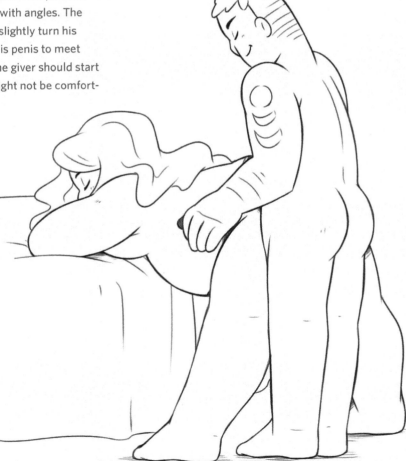

Pull Up to the Bumper

The receiver is on her knees on the seat of a couch, with her hands gripping its back. The giver stands behind her in between her legs and enters. From here, either the giver or the receiver can control the ride—the giver by gripping the receiver's hips or waist, and the receiver by pushing off the couch with her arms and knees.

Elle's Big Girl Move

Both participants can take an active role thrusting, making a usually submissive position for the receiver more dominant (if she wishes). Power dynamic can also be played with here—the giver can remain still and the receiver can use her leverage to pump backward onto his cock. Also, the giver's hands are free to fondle her boobs, or to reach around the receiver to her clit, or to spread her butt cheeks and play with the entrance to her anus.

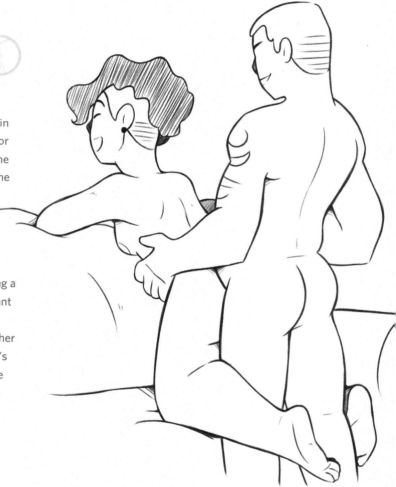

Bunny Rabbit

The receiver kneels on the edge of the bed with legs spread and lowers her butt to her heels. The giver stands behind her and enters. The giver can use his hands to spread the receiver's butt cheeks if more room is needed for entry. Once things get going, those hands can move to the receiver's hips, providing the giver with the control he needs to thrust like a bunny. If it's more comfortable for either partner, the receiver can bend forward and place her forearms on the bed while the giver can place his torso on her back.

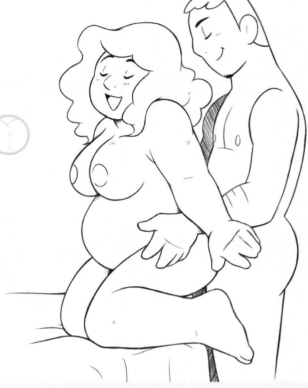

Porn Sex vs. Realistic Sex

Chances are that if you own a computer you've seen some porn. Porn can be empowering and arousing to look at, but it's important not to confuse porn sex with the style of sex that people around the world have every day. Porn actors (who are essentially sex athletes) are positioned for the best camera angles, and their movements are choreographed to heighten sexual entertainment. Foreplay, impromptu body noises, muscle tweaks, and the like are condensed or edited out. Porn is *not* an instruction manual for how people do or must have sex in their everyday lives or how they must look in order to have passionate, fulfilling, hot sex—it's for visual stimulation only.

Sidewinder

The receiver lies on her side with her leg closest to the bed extended straight and the other knee pulled to her chest (or as close to her chest as possible). The giver straddles her extended leg on his knees, aligns the genitals, and enters. The giver can thrust while leaning over (or winding around) their partner. The receiver shouldn't be shy to adjust a larger tummy or hold back a butt cheek. The Sidewinder gives both partners a unique angle for penetration for a refreshing change.

Soap Is the Kryptonite of the Vulva

Your vulva is a perfect biome for healthy bacteria (lactobacilli) that live there. Washing the inside of your vulva with soap disturbs the delicate ecosystem that keeps your vulva healthy. Soap kills the good bacteria in your vulva, giving the bad bacteria an opportunity to move in and grow. The disruption of pH in the vulva may cause an unusual smell (anywhere from ammonia to dead fish), which is sometimes an indication of vaginitis, bacterial vaginosis (BV), or a yeast infection.

In short, your vulva is self-cleaning, so stick to washing the outside of your vulva (labia majora) or rinsing the inside of your vulva with hot water and you should be just fine. If you want to feel clean without soap, look for products made for that delicate area that state they have a "neutral pH" (see Curvy Resources, page 178). This kind of cleanser generally won't kill the essential bacteria on your vulva.

The Iron Throne

The receiver stands behind her Iron Throne (a chair, preferably—not one made of swords), and then leans over the chair's back. The giver enters from behind. The features of the chair can be used to heighten the experience: If it has arms, the receiver can hold on tight, or if the back is low, she can bend over farther to get down and dirty. And if the chair is really sturdy, the receiver can relax into it while the giver pumps intensely. Soon, winter won't be the only thing that's coming!

Elle's Big Girl Move

One of my favorite things in the world is hotel sex. You're someplace new, you don't have to make the bed, people can make and bring you meals, and you have an array of new furnishings just begging for you to have sex on them! Next time you're looking to book a room, check out the photos first. You know you'll get a bed, but note that armless chairs, stools, and ottomans are versatile for all different kinds of sex positions in this book. Is there a big window strong enough to lean against for some upright lovin'? Is there a sofa? A desk? A shower with a built-in bench? And here's an expert tip: Request that extra pillows and towels be put in your room prior to arrival. You'll thank me later.

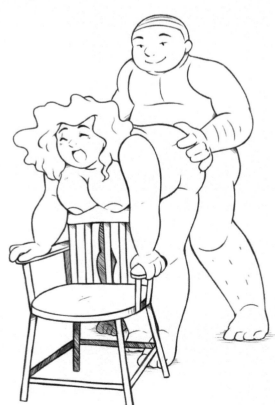

The Rock Star

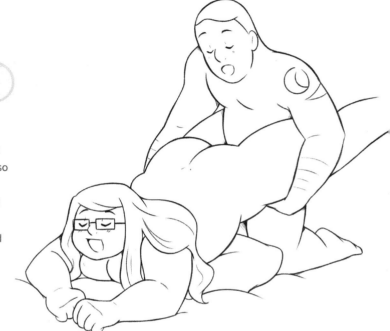

In this one, the giver gets to channel their inner David Bowie, to rock out with their . . . well, you get the idea. On her knees, the receiver spreads her legs and rests her torso and hips on a stack of firm pillows or cushions. The giver is on his knees between the receiver's legs. He enters and lifts one of her legs up and out to the side. The receiver can hold on to the pillows underneath her for stability and control. The giver can use the elevated leg for thrusting leverage, and holds on to a hip with the other hand, or he can bring both hands to the elevated leg for a bit of impromptu, mid-sex air guitar!

Sex Positivity

If you haven't come across the term "sex-positive" yet, here is a quick overview. As society becomes more aware of varying sexual practices, genders, and sexualities, people who support, advocate for, and understand that sexuality is a positive and inalienable right are considered "sex-positive." Sex positivity veers away from common negative beliefs about sex—for example, that sex is shameful or a marital duty. Being sex-positive means that (among other things) you believe that safe, consensual, enjoyable, judgment-free sex should be encouraged in your life and for others. But it's also important to note that part of sex positivity is accepting and supporting people (including yourself) who don't want to have sex at a particular time or at all. If you believe that shame-free, safe, consensual sex for yourself (and others) is something you believe in, that's sex-positive.

Flying Wheelbarrow

For this advanced position, the receiver starts on hands and knees. The giver then lifts her legs, allowing her to wrap them around his waist and to hook her ankles behind his back. The giver can bend his knees for extra stability and leverage.

Elle's Big Girl Move

This is a position that can be used to the receiver's advantage when experimenting with different pieces of furniture. A high or long ottoman would work just as well as a bed. With an ottoman, the receiver might be able to hold on to one end or grasp the sides for more stability. Also, if it's not possible or comfortable to wrap legs and lock ankles around your partner, don't. Adjust this position to be most comfortable for you. If the receiver's lower back aches, just place a pillow under her hips to ease arch pressure.

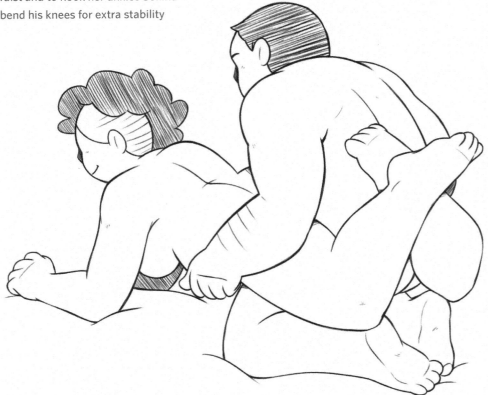

Leapfrog

     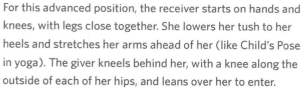

For this advanced position, the receiver starts on hands and knees, with legs close together. She lowers her tush to her heels and stretches her arms ahead of her (like Child's Pose in yoga). The giver kneels behind her, with a knee along the outside of each of her hips, and leans over her to enter.

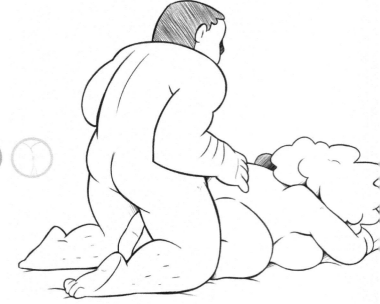

Elle's Big Girl Move

Sex from behind is great in general for the dominant and submissive in either of you. However, the Leapfrog is especially fun if the giver wants to really take control. In this position, the giver has free range to grab the receiver's hips and really plunge with vigor and passion. If the receiver puts her arms back and to the side, the giver can hold her hands while thrusting and controlling the receiver's movement. You can try putting a pillow underneath the receiver's hips to augment the receiver's pitch and offer both partners an alternate sensation.

Slip 'n' Slide

The receiver lies face down on the bed while the giver applies massage oil to the entire back of her body. The giver then lies on top of the receiver and uses his whole body to massage his partner. The giver can experiment with different ways to move against his partner while the receiver relaxes and enjoys the body worship showered upon her and concentrates on the range of sensations created by connecting with the whole body.

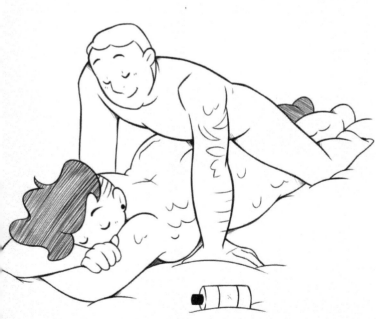

Elle's Big Girl Move

The Slip 'n' Slide position was inspired by the Japanese erotic art of Nuru massage. In Japan, the Nuru massage was named for the body-to-body erotic massage that originated in the bath-houses of Japan called "soaplands." A Nuru massage is traditionally facilitated using a natural, non-staining, clear slippery gel made out of nori, a seaweed extract. Using a very large, stationary, rubber or plastic air mattress shaped like a box (to keep you from sliding into the next room), practitioners sit with their client on the mattress, while they cover each other in gel. The client lays down flat, while the practitioner climbs on top and slides, rubs, glides, and undulates on top of the client, "massaging" the client with her body. Hot, right?

You don't even have to go all the way to Japan to have a Nuru massage. There are companies that make Nuru massage kits to bring home and turn any room in your house into a slippery massage parlor (see Curvy Resources, page 178). All you need to do is set up a sexy and seductive atmosphere. Remember to have plenty of towels around the outside of the massage area to step in and out so you don't slip and fall. Before you begin, ask your sweetheart to take a shower with you and wash him (and yourself) well before you lead him into the massage area. Then, let the games begin!

Chapter

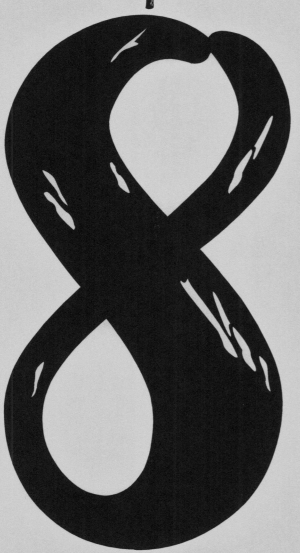

Strapping it on as a fat femme makes me feel sexy, aroused, and empowered, especially if I really dress myself up, putting on heels, red lipstick, and thigh-high fishnets, which attach to the garter belt built into my harness. I love the gender variation of my feminine curves with the masculine cock I'm wearing, and that contrast is not only what gets me off; it's the reminder that my curves are beautiful, sensual, and worthy of worship (just like your curves are!).

Lauren Marie Fleming, author of
Bawdy Love: 10 Steps to Profoundly
Loving Your Body

Spooning, Scissoring, and

SIDEWAYS SEX

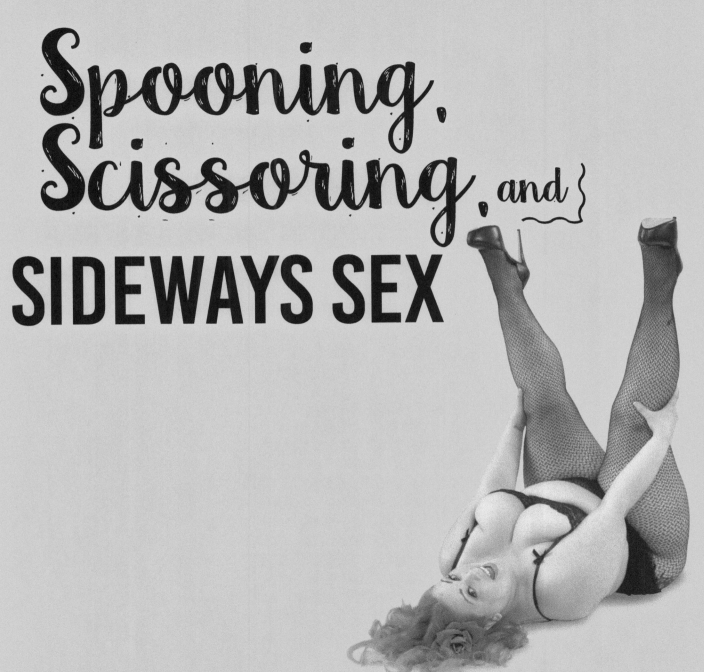

Spooning, scissoring, and sideways sex can be challenging for those of us with shapely butts and thicker thighs, or with a partner who has a larger stomach.

However, for all of its possible angles and poses, sex sideways can also be one of the most versatile. Manipulating angles can give both partners the opportunity to see each other better, as well as relish a handful of hip or a bouncing breast. After checking out these nine sideways-inspired positions (or while you're test-driving them), think about ways you can improve upon them for the comfort and thrill of your unique body and that of your partner's.

Spooning and sideways positions can get hot and dirty but they also can be about building connection and closeness. If you want to get super intimate and close, sideways sex can get deep quick when you're skin-to-skin against your lover and moving in rhythm together. Your bodies feel snug and more conjoined than ever.

Another reason that the sideways situations are terrific is that this is an angle that the vagina doesn't always get to feel. You may find that inserting a penis or dildo at certain sideways or scissoring angles stimulates a part of the vaginal canal you never knew could feel so good!

As if the benefits of these positions couldn't get any better, the following poses also ensure one or both of your hands are free to massage a scalp, rub a pussy, play with a breast, or grip all the parts you adore on your lover. So go forth and spoon!

Flower Bud

Begin by spooning, with the receiver as the little spoon. The receiver wraps her top leg around the giver's thigh as the giver props himself up with his lower elbow and enters. He can use his top hand to stimulate her vulva, clitoris, or nipple to coax her flower to bloom.

You Are Not Your Body

If your partner wasn't turned on by you they wouldn't be having sex with you. That's just a fact. A lot of curvy girls can feel self-conscious, uncomfortably vulnerable, or just plain scared to engage in a position like the Flower Bud where their tummy is so exposed. This is a good time to re-train your mind away from the self-effacing or worrisome thoughts that might be coming up for you. A great way to do this is to not beat yourself up for feeling or thinking the way you do. Instead, notice you're having the thought, acknowledge it in your mind, and then replace that thought by focusing on the pleasure you're receiving and giving.

Use all your senses. Listen to your partner's breathing (or moaning) and see if you can determine his/her level of pleasure by its changing patterns. Hone in on body language and movements and how they communicate arousal. Concentrate on what it feels like where all the parts of your skin connect. Ask yourself what feels good, what's just okay, and what is incredibly arousing. Stop the negative thoughts by focusing on what's happening in the moment and on what kind of pleasure you can or are giving your partner, then revel in your ability to be present and in your pleasure at the same time as your partner—that's no small feat!

Open Flower

Begin by spooning, with the receiver as the little spoon.
The receiver raises her top leg in the air, opening herself up
like a flower. The giver supports the lifted leg with his hand
and enters. The receiver can stimulate herself manually or
with a vibrator. If butt cheeks or thighs get in the way, the
giver can bring her leg up toward her chest and the giver
can use his free hand to manipulate her cheeks or thighs
away from the genitals.

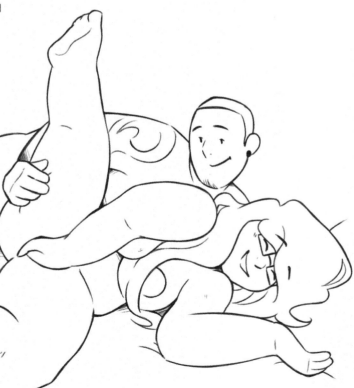

Spooning

Begin by spooning with the receiver as the little spoon. Tilting forward, the receiver opens her legs slightly to allow better access to the genitals for the giver to enter. From here the giver can use his outside hand to stimulate the breasts or clitoris, grip the hips for greater thrusting leverage, or spread the butt cheeks to allow deeper penetration or clearer access.

"People in fat bodies are taught by our society that we already take up too much physical space. We are expected to take what we can get, to accept pity, to play small lest someone notice us. Because of that, too many of us don't know how to advocate for ourselves in the bedroom. We feel ashamed if we need extra pillows or a special ramp to make a position comfortable. We try to hide the fact that we're out of breath or not as limber as our partner. All of that takes away from our pleasure. The truth is that every single lover I've had has eagerly accommodated any changes I needed to be more comfortable or relaxed. It hasn't been easy, but as soon as I started asking for what I needed, sex took on a whole new dimension. My fat body? It's pretty phenomenal at pleasure and orgasms. I just had to find my voice and the rest fell into place."

Dawn Serra, sex coach

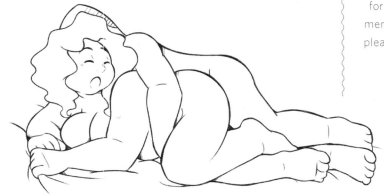

When Penetration Is Uncomfortable

Most of the nerve endings that give you pleasure are located within the first 2 inches (5 cm) or so of the vaginal opening. Some vaginas enjoy the feeling of deep penetration, but some do not. In fact, some find it irritating if the penis or dildo thrusts fast and deep and hits the cervix. If deep penetration isn't fun for you, don't fret. Try one of these solutions:

- If your partner's penis or dildo is on the longer side, try inserting a shorter dildo to see if it feels more comfortable. Let your partner know that using his entire length during sex is uncomfortable/painful.

- Use more lube.
- Slow down the giver's pace if it's too vigorous.
- Rest and come back to penetrative sex another time. You may simply be more sensitive, or your cervix (which can move depending on time of the month) may be in a vulnerable position.

If you are in pain at any time, stop. If the issue continues, see your healthcare provider to make certain there isn't anything out of whack.

Nesting Bird

In this advanced position, both partners lie on their sides facing each other. The receiver pulls her top knee to her chest, allowing her shin to settle on the giver's chest or under his arm, thereby opening up the pelvic region and allowing a generous area for her partner to enter. Both partners can wrap their top arm around the other, giving them the ability to grasp each other as they thrust and grind. If they are too far apart to do that comfortably, the receiver can reach between them and stimulate her clitoris, and the giver can reach her breasts. Or they can both grasp each other's arms for thrusting leverage and control.

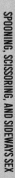

Scissoring

Scissoring (also called tribadism) is essentially nonpenetrative sex between two vulvas. The two partners can assume the position pictured, or variations of it depending on body types, sizes, and comfort levels. Sometimes adding a wand vibrator to the mix can make both clits happy at the same time. One partner holds the head of the wand between both partners' clits, while both of you grind against it and use each other as leverage. A wand vibe can be essential for two larger partners who want to get off this way. If you want the feeling of penetration, a double-ended dildo, like the Fun Factory Share or the Tantus Feel-Doe are ideal and come in different sizes with the option of vibration. If folds and flesh are determined to foil plans, try scissoring while both partners lie down, with each of you grasping hands (or ankles) to gain more power to push against each other and create delicious friction.

"There's no such thing as the 'right' way to have girl-on-girl sex. Experimentation, languid exploration, and fierce connection are all part of the game. So try new positions, new toys, new dynamics knowing that girl sex is all about the fun you can have together!"

Allison Moon,
author of *Girl Sex 101*

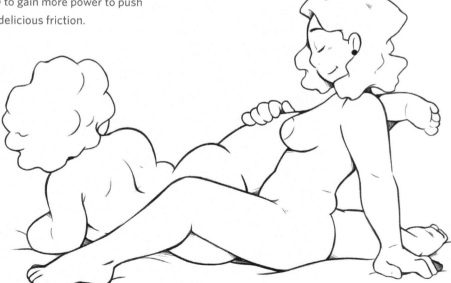

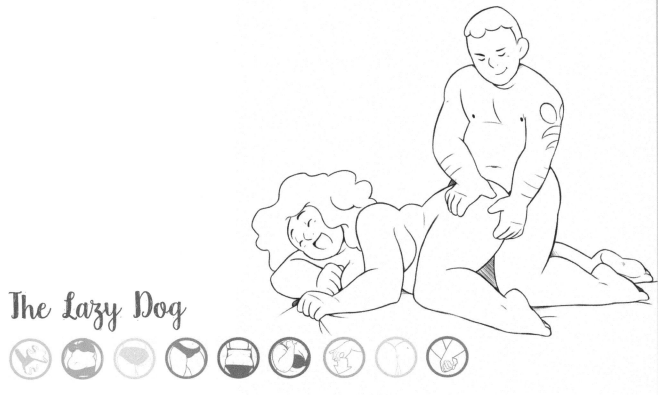

The Lazy Dog

The receiver lies on her side, with legs straight. Bending her top knee, she rests it on the bed in front of her. On his knees, the giver straddles the receiver's straight leg at the thigh and enters. The giver can use the receiver's top hip for balance or more controlled thrusting. He can also use his hands to spread the receiver's butt cheeks for deeper penetration. If it's more comfortable or provides better access, the receiver can elevate her bent leg by placing a pillow underneath it or, for more limber lovers, raising the bent knee and placing the flat of her foot on the bed right in front of her. The receiver can hold back or push aside a larger stomach for more range of motion.

Elle's Big Girl Move

As is, the angle of this position doesn't give easy access for clitoral stimulation. However, clit stimulation can be achieved by the receiver exposing the vulva by either manipulating the flesh of the upper butt cheek and thigh or lifting up her outer leg so that the clit is more easily accessible for the giver to stimulate with his free hand. He can then massage the clit manually or use a bullet vibe or strong vibrating wand on the clit to get her off as he rides her into orgasmic nirvana.

Winding Vine

You will never look at ivy the same way again! In the Winding Vine, both partners are on their sides and facing each other, arms intertwined. The receiver wraps her top leg over the giver's top leg, giving him room to enter. The giver can hold on to the wrapped leg for thrusting power, or the receiver can wrap it tightly and do some thrusting of her own. If tummies are making this position challenging, create a gap between your chests and pull the tummy flesh up to clear the way. Once penetration is achieved, get closer again to pin your tummies together and out of the way.

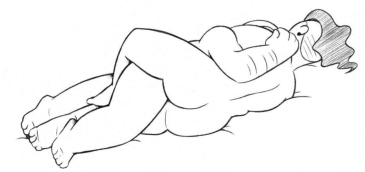

Getting Hot from Getting Cool

Studies suggest that your sex drive decreases in the warm summer months, so take a fresh approach to foreplay when it's hot outside. Why not wash the car on a hot day and get playful with the hose? Catch a summer blockbuster in the cool, dark movie theater. Use your time wisely by fondling your partner's inner thighs, grazing your fingers lightly over (or under) those clothes, offer light kisses on the neck or inside the wrists—think sensual instead of sexual. Pay less attention to your partner's sweet spot and more on a range of erogenous zones. By the time the movie is over, you'll be itching to get home and tear each other's clothes off.

The Spork

The giver lies on his side while the receiver lies on her back with her legs draped over the giver's hips so that their genitals are aligned. The receiver opens her legs slightly to allow the giver to enter. The giver may prop himself up with his bottom arm while his top arm remains free to stimulate her breasts or clitoris. The receiver's hands are free to caress her parts or spread her butt cheeks to allow for deeper penetration.

"Some of us are just lucky to have an inner core of confidence that has no clear genesis. It just exists. But even women who aren't so lucky to be somehow born with the 'I feel sexy' gene, seem to be able to learn to feel sexy. The key is listening and believing when you are told you are attractive and that someone is attracted to you. . . . The ones telling us the truth are sharing our beds and our hearts. It is them we must believe. . . . When you feel sexy, you project sexy, and others find you sexy. It's not so important how you get there, but that you get there."

**Rebecca Jane Weinstein,
lawyer, social worker, and author of
*Fat Sex: The Naked Truth***

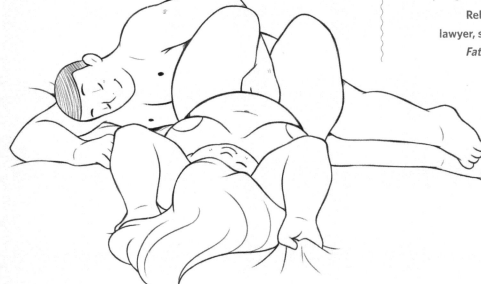

Myth: Fat Girls are Easy

As if *easy* is a bad thing! This myth typically implies that "fat chicks" are promiscuous because sex is the only way they can get someone to go out with them. Not only is this idea offensive, it's born from the insecurity, bigotry, and low self-esteem of the speaker. We know that making broad assumptions about anyone's sexuality, gender, political affiliations, religious or spiritual beliefs, or heritage is not just inaccurate, but wrong. Why should someone's size be any different? As long as you're not hurting yourself or others, there's nothing wrong with having sex as many times and with as many people as you please. This myth also suggests that being "easy" is "slutty" and therefore an insult as well, and that's called "slut shaming." If you find yourself being slut-shamed by anyone, sex coach and author Charlie Glickman, Ph.D., suggests this simple response: "I'm not easy, I'm selectively convenient." Then drop your imaginary mic and walk away.

The Sideways Ohm

This is a favorite for the range of vaginal sensations it provides *plus* unlimited clit access! The receiver lies on her side, with her knees bent in front of her. On his knees, the giver places himself directly behind the receiver's bum and enters. From here, he can hold on to her hip to assist with balance or for greater leverage when thrusting. He can also use his hands to spread her butt cheeks to allow for deeper or clearer entry. The receiver can then lift her outer leg up as he thrusts to try a variety of angles to experience new sensations, or revisit one that you know makes your toes curl.

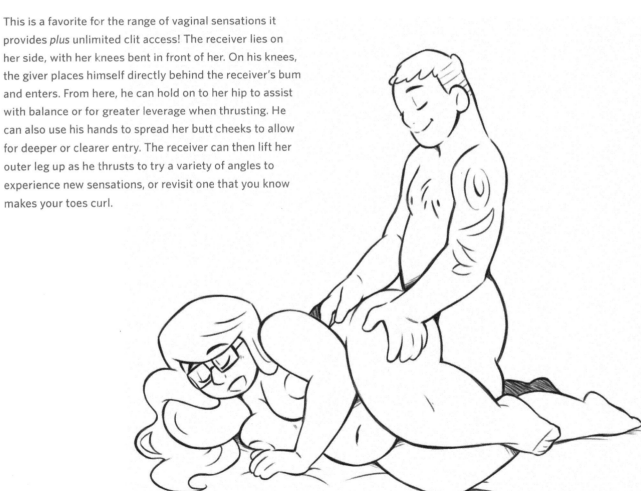

Chapter

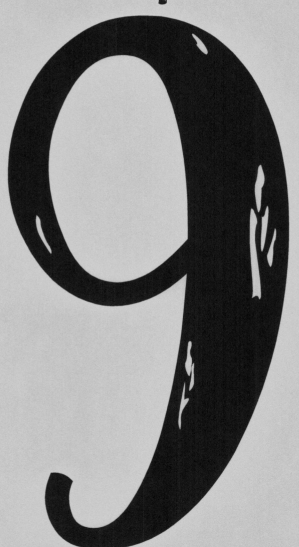

Just because you're in penetrative-sex-land doesn't mean you have to keep going till one or both of you come. That's the way your grandma had sex. Change up your patterns! Surprise each other! Hop off and go down, playfully tickle and lick, tease and admire each other. Until one of you says "Don't stop, please don't stop," it's all still on the table.

Sex Nerd Sandra, humorist, sex educator, podcaster

Oral and Hand SEX

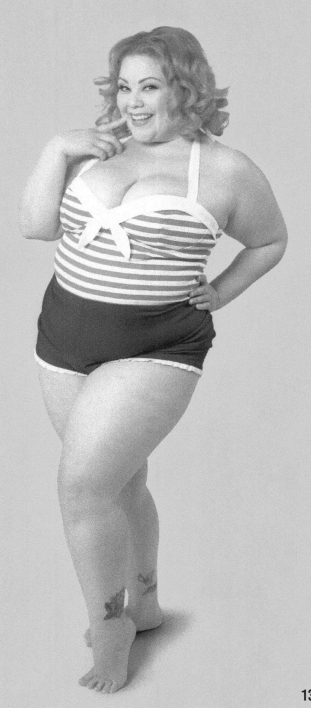

Oral sex is one of the most intimate sex acts you can take part in, and in many ways it can feel more intimate than penetrative sex.

It is a vulnerable act in which you relinquish control of your most private and sensitive body part to your partner. It requires trust. You're allowing this person to lavish your vulva, clit, and vagina with attention. Knowing that your lover enjoys supping on you creates a unique connection and intimacy.

The same goes for hand sex. Sometimes called "mutual masturbation," hand sex is manual stimulation of the genitals— inserting fingers in the vagina or ass, or rubbing your partner's clit with your fingers. Hand sex can be thrilling when done covertly under the table at a restaurant, to profoundly deep when naked, facing each other, and incredibly aroused.

Depending on body size and shape, getting into position for comfortable oral or hand sex can be easy or arduous. But here's a variety of positions for oral and hand sex that will make these tasks easy and fun for both of you. Let's take a tour, shall we?

The Gift

This is the instinctive oral-sex receiver position that most people end up trying first. Traditionally, the receiver lies back on the bed, with her legs spread and her knees bent and pointing upward. The giver places his face between her spread legs to provide oral, or his hands to provide manual stimulation. For those of us with fleshy tummies, hips, or thighs, propping up the hips with several firm pillows (or a Liberator Wedge) will draw our flowy parts back, opening up the designated area for oral action and presenting the vulva like the gift it is.

Elle's Big Girl Move

Sometimes, those of us with larger lower bellies that may hang in front of the mons have concerns about access and breathing room while our partners are performing oral sex. But no need to fear! I have a hack or two. After the receiver props up her hips, she can reach forward to press her mons down, or down and back (whichever she prefers), while the giver sidles up to perform oral sex. This should create plenty of room for the giver to breathe comfortably.

If that doesn't quite do it, the receiver should use her fingers to spread her labial folds, giving her partner direct access. In fact, using this technique actually creates an airway between your partner's nose and your hand.

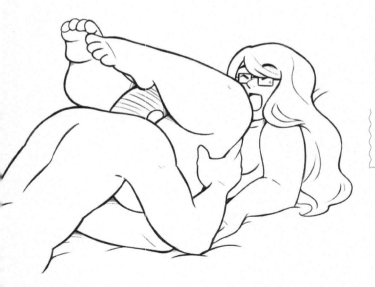

The Harp

The receiver lies on her back. The giver lies on her side next to her to provide manual stimulation and enjoy the view. This is a great position for your lover to lavish attention on you and your beautiful body. Lie back and revel in the sensation of your partner stimulating you while she whispers erotic nothings into your ear in between passionate kisses. Is it hot in here?

Take a Deep Breath

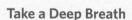

When I'm asked what the number-one tip for better sex is, I always say conscious breathing. By controlling your breath, you also control the oxygen in your bloodstream. Highly oxygenated blood gives our bodies more energy and helps our organs function to their highest potential. Just learning how to do one very simple specific breathing technique—like Breath of Fire or synchronized breathing with your partner—during

sex and at climax can significantly improve your pleasure in the moment. Also, concentrating on your breath keeps you focused on what is happening in the moment and is a great way to distract your mind from any negative thoughts that might come up. You can learn more on this topic by reading *Urban Tantra* by Barbara Carrellas and *The Multi-Orgasmic Man* by Mantak Chia and Douglas Abrams.

Suppertime

Dinner is served! The receiver positions herself by lying back on a table, with her tush close to the edge. The giver pulls up a seat, places the receiver's legs on her shoulders, and enjoys the dish. Depending on table height, the giver may forgo a chair and opt to kneel. This position is fantastic for curvy gals and their lovers because the giver's hands are free to manipulate body parts or skin out of the way if needed, and can still use a free hand to place a finger (or more) inside the vagina to stimulate the G-spot.

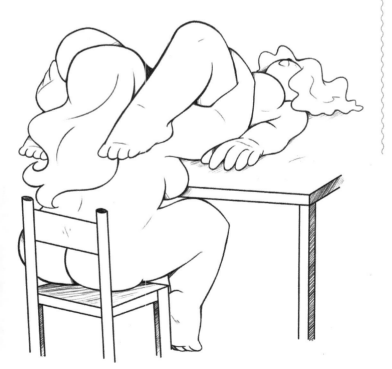

"Big girls typically don't feel like they deserve to be sexy. Fat shaming has taken away our right to take up sexy space in fishnets, bodysuits, baby dolls, and thigh highs. And it's harder to shop for these things as a big girl. We fight the challenge of finding clothing that fits *and* looks good on our bodies, but also feeling like we look good with bellies, thighs that touch, arms that jiggle, and breasts that sag. I love how lingerie makes me feel. It is decorating my sexiness and alluring both my partner and me to inspire lust."

Luna Matatas, burlesque performer, sex and pleasure educator

Amuse-Bouche

An amuse-bouche is a "little taste," but your partner will want more than a little in this sexy stance! Standing beside the bed with her legs spread, the receiver bends forward and lowers her torso onto the mattress, resting her weight on her forearms. The giver kneels on the floor between the receiver's legs and proceeds to "dine" on the feast in front of him. The receiver has the option to remain passive and enjoy, or actively move her hips to help direct where she wants to be stimulated.

Elle's Big Girl Move

If a larger bottom half makes access to the goods a little challenging for the giver, the receiver can bend one knee to the side and rest it on the bed. This will open up her genital area for the giver, and if the receiver has a sore back, it can alleviate some pressure on the lower lumbar.

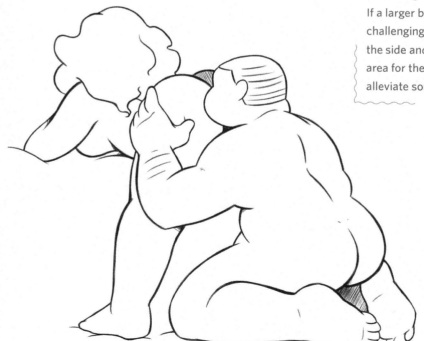

69

Ah, 69—the equal-opportunity position. Everyone gives and everyone receives in this position made for mutual oral pleasure. One partner lies on his back, and, facing his genitals, the other kneels or crouches to straddle his face. The partner on top leans forward to bring her face to her partner's nether region. Once in place, both partners can orally or manually stimulate each other. This is great for curvy girls because the bottom partner's hands are free to maneuver bellies or thighs, if needed.

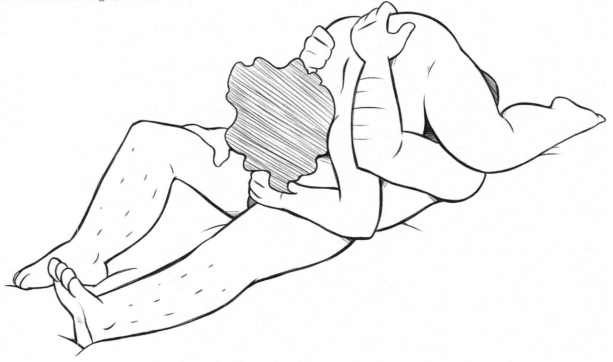

96

This is another take on 69 that some curvy gals find more comfortable. For simultaneous oral stimulation fun without anyone being the bottom or the top, try 96. In this fun dual-pleaser, partners lie on their sides facing each another. Each partner's head is aligned with the other's genitals, allowing for convenient oral (and manual) delight.

Elle's Big Girl Move

Different variations of 96 can soothe sore wrists, necks, or backs and leave a hand free to move flesh out of the way. For instance, partners can rest their head on each other's bottom legs for a more mellow, relaxing experience—and freeing up at least one arm, which can be laid across the anterior hip for anal or vaginal play. Even better, each partner can bend the anterior leg, placing her foot on the bed and opening up the thighs for an easier means of approach and more stabilization for the body.

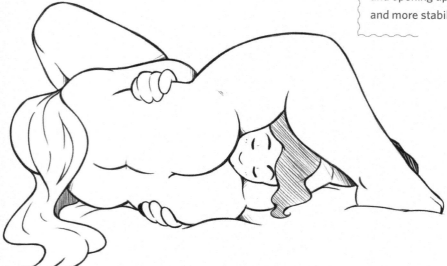

The Coronation

For this twist on 69, the receiver lies on her back on the
floor, but close to a wall, with her butt facing the wall
and her legs straight up in the air. Bending her knees and
spreading her legs, she slides her feet down the wall half-
way, as if she were going to push it with her feet. The giver,
facing the same wall, kneels and straddles the receiver's
head, and then leans forward to provide oral stimulation.
The receiver has the option of returning the oral favor,
providing manual stimulation, or simply lying back and
enjoying herself. Long live the queen!

Yin Yang

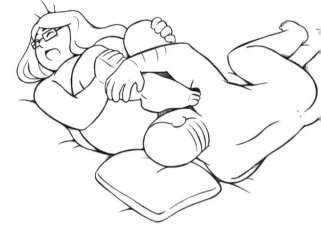

The receiver lies on her back with her knees pulled toward her chest. With his head supported by a pillow, the giver lies perpendicular to her, with his face at her vulva. From here, the giver can provide manual or oral stimulation (and enjoy the view). This is a great position for your lover to lavish attention on you and your beautiful body. Lie back and revel in the sensation of your partner stimulating you while she whispers erotic nothings into your ear in between passionate kisses. Is it hot in here?

Hot Dam!

Remember that oral sex is still sex, meaning there are bodily fluids involved. Though contracting an STI via oral sex is considered lower risk, there is still a risk, and as such, I suggest using some sort of barrier method (e.g., condom, dental dam) when giving or receiving head. For people with vulvas, dental dams are the barrier method of choice for cunnilingus. Made out of a large rectangle of extremely thin but strong latex, these swathes of rubber come plain or in different flavors, such as licorice, cola, and strawberry. To use a dam during oral sex, the giver stretches the dam over the vulva (and anus if need be) while pleasuring her lover. If you or your sweetie are allergic to latex, you can order nonlatex (usually nitrile or polyisoprene) dental dams from a dental supply site. In a pinch, you can always cut one side of a nonlatex condom or glove and use that instead.

Checking the Oil

A good mechanic will always check the oil, and so should your partner. The receiver gets on hands and knees, like in the Doggy Style position (page 103). The giver kneels by her side and provides manual stimulation to the clitoris, vulva, and breasts.

Elle's Big Girl Move

This versatile and highly erotic position lends itself to a few styles of play. A super sultry change of pace is to take it into the world of sensual massage. The giver asks the receiver to get into position (with pillows underneath her torso for support, if need be) and proceeds to rub massage oil on the receiver's back, behind, and back of the legs avoiding all the places she's expecting to be touched. The giver proceeds to massage the oil into his partner's skin slowly and sensually, maybe stopping along the way to kiss her neck, whisper something salacious in her ear, or play with her hair. He may gradually begin to oil up the heretofore neglected body parts of the receiver, like the breasts, tummy, and inside of the thighs, saving the best body part for last. By the time the giver gets to the vulva and clit, the receiver might be ready to explode, so proceed with caution and watch your lover melt into the bed.

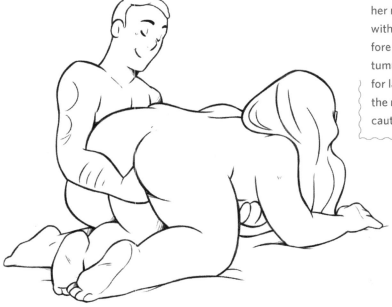

Rubbing the Lantern

Get ready to feel like the center of the universe with this hand-sex favorite. The receiver lies back with her legs spread, knees bent, and hips supported by pillows. The giver sits between her legs and luxuriously massages the vulva and clitoris; with his other hand, he can stroke her thighs or tummy, or gratify himself at the same time! As clitoral sensitivity may vary, be sure to check in to ensure that the receiver is enjoying her massage.

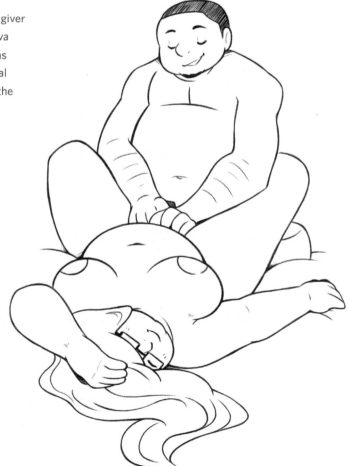

Sanskrit, Schmanskrit: What's a Yoni?

Rubbing the Lantern is inspired by what Tantra practitioners call a "Yoni massage." In Sanskrit, Yoni means the vulva or "sacred space." A Yoni massage is a slow and methodical worshipping of the receiver's vulva, the area around it and inside of the labial folds. This can be a transformative act for partners who wish to deepen the intimacy in a relationship or as a way to relax the receiver enough so that they can fully enjoy the pleasure being given to them.

In a Yoni massage there is no goal other than to give or receive sensual pleasure; the receiver should not feel any expectation or pressure to orgasm, but should approach this Yoni massage with reverence, sensitivity, and no expectation of reciprocation. The giver should tune into their partner and take notice of breathing patterns, moans, and body language for cues as to where

and how she is receiving the most pleasure and what kind of touch she likes most. The receiver should set the intention to relax and receive the pleasure being given to her. She should spend this time focusing on how good her partner's fingers, hands, warmth, and movements feel on her vulva. She should take notice of her process of arousal, wetness, breathing, and how her body is moving instinctively.

At the end of the Yoni massage, check in with your partner and discuss what you both liked about the exercise and anything you might have learned or noticed about your arousal process and your body. You might find that you've discovered something about yourself sensually that you didn't know before, which is its own gift.

Yes, No, Maybe

What do you do if you want to try sexy new things with your partner, but don't know where to start? Where do you begin if you're about to become sexual with a new partner and want to make certain you both know each other's sexual boundaries? Try a "Yes, No, Maybe" list. This is a comprehensive checklist of potential sexual acts that people can engage in (e.g., finger in butt, light hair pulling, role play, spanking). Next to each act there is a space to note whether that act is a "yes" (I'd like to do this), "no" (I will never do this), or "maybe" (I might do this at some point). A "no" is considered a "hard limit," which by definition is an act that is *non-negotiable* or a firm boundary. A "maybe" is considered a "soft limit," meaning that it's something that could be considered at some point or might be negotiable. Regardless, an act that is a "maybe" needs to be discussed, and terms agreed upon by both partners, before engaging in it. If the "maybe" hasn't been discussed, and boundaries and rules haven't been accepted and agreed upon in advance, consider it a "no" until that discussion occurs.

What if you're interested in a little light bondage but are sheepish about bringing it up with your partner? Introduce the yes, no, maybe list to your partner like this: Print out two copies of the list (download it free from www.ellechase.com) and mention to your partner that you think it might make your fabulous sex life more intimate, adventurous, or exciting if you shared some likes, dislikes, and possibilities for sex play that you haven't tried yet. Both of you should fill it out separately and compare it to see how you match up. This will certainly get the conversation and/or negotiation started. Even if you end up trying just a couple of things or nothing at all, you've done something new and different to improve your communication, intimacy, and sex life. So pat yourself on the back—you went outside your comfort zone and that takes a lot of courage!

Captive Audience

The receiver sits in a chair with her legs spread and butt close to the front of the seat. The giver kneels in front of her to perform cunnilingus. If the giver's hands aren't busy stroking her vulva, they can be stimulating her clit, pushing a tummy aside for more access, or pleasuring himself. So many options!

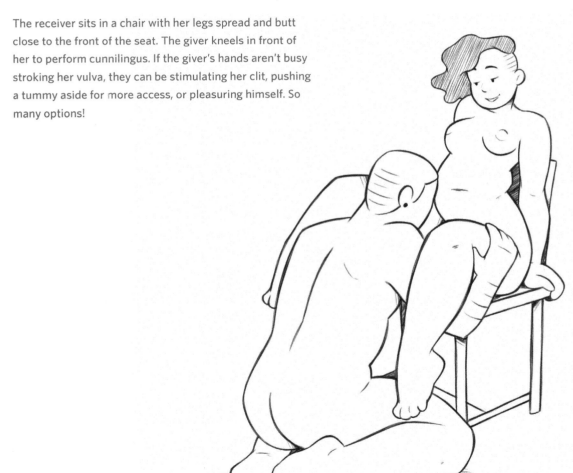

Doorknocker

The receiver is on her hands and knees. The giver kneels behind her, lowering his chest to rest on her back. From here the giver is free to stimulate the breasts, genitals, or anus with his hands. Because of how the bodies are aligned in the Doorknocker, this position lends itself to some frottage. If the giver feels like it, he can rub his genitals against her bum and vulva while he stimulates her with his fingers. The Doorknocker can also feel very sensual and intimate with both of your bodies being so close together. And if things get hot and heavy, you're both in a perfect position for rear entry, just remember to have lube and condoms at the ready!

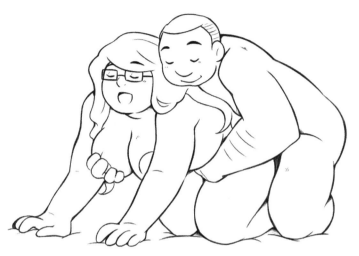

The Silicone Hand Jive

We've talked about the necessity for lube during penetrative sex in Chapter 2, but hand sex is no exception. Often, hand sex can be a precursor to penetrative sex. Hand sex during foreplay can help get the receiver turned on, wet, and ready for accepting a penis or dildo. But the receiver is not always sufficiently lubricated when hand is put to vulva. Using a personal lubricant meant for the sensitive genital area is important when trying to stimulate or penetrate a partner with hands

or a toy. For hand sex, I recommend a premium silicone lube like Sliquid Silver, which has only three ingredients. Sometimes called a glide, silicone lube sits on top of the skin, as opposed to being absorbed, and therefore lasts longer than water-based lube. You can also use a food-grade oil, like coconut oil. If using a toy, the safe bet is a water-based or silk hybrid, because straight silicone lube will break down the material of a silicone toy and make it sticky and unusable.

The Ambigram

In this advanced position, one partner starts on her hands and knees while the other partner slides underneath her, aligning each other's heads with genitals. The top partner straightens her arms and legs, coming into Downward Dog (see page 106). From this position, both partners can engage in stimulation. The top partner can orally stimulate the bottom, and the bottom partner can manually stimulate the top partner. Everybody wins!

Elle's Big Girl Move

If getting into Downward Dog is uncomfortable for the partner on top, she can rest on her knees instead, effectively straddling the bottom partner's head while supporting herself on her forearms on either side of the bottom partner's hips. This also gives the bottom partner the choice to orally or manually stimulate the top partner, or just sit back and enjoy the view.

Polishing the Silver

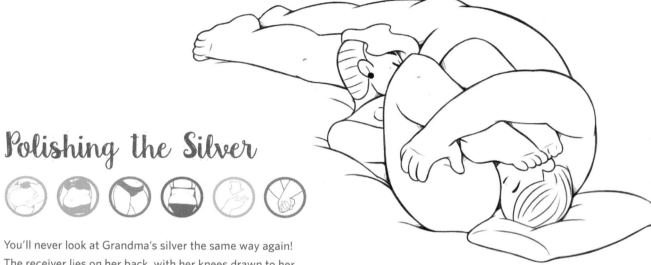

You'll never look at Grandma's silver the same way again! The receiver lies on her back, with her knees drawn to her chest. The giver lies next to her on his opposite side, with his head facing the receiver's genitals so he can sup. The giver can place his anterior arm over the receiver's bent legs, holding them in place, or can use his hand to push aside the buttocks and thigh to make access to the honey pot even sweeter. Since the partners are positioned so their faces are aligned with each other's genitals, the receiver might have enough reach to engage in manual stimulation on herself or her partner.

Elle's Big Girl Move

If the giver has a penis, this is a fun position for a toy called a male masturbator. Masturbators usually come as a hollow, cylindrical sleeve made out of a soft, fleshlike material, though some can come in the shape of a hollow egg, flat like a pancake to be wrapped around the penis, or encased in a hard plastic housing. The inside of the masturbators can be smooth, but are often textured to give more sensation for the user. To use one, coat the inside of the sleeve and/or the penis with a water-based lube, slip the penis inside the sleeve, and stroke away. The combination of the soft silicone, lube, motion, warmth, and grip of the hand gives the penis the feeling of penetrating a real vagina, ass, or mouth. A masturbation sleeve is great to have around if you have a partner with a penis and enjoy mutual masturbation, or to add something new and different to a hand job or a blow job to give your mouth a break.

Queen for a Day

This is a classic queening position that some givers (and receivers) find intensely erotic. *Queening* is any position in which the receiver straddles the giver's face to receive oral sex. The giver lies flat on his back while the receiver squats over or straddles his head. From here, the giver can massage the receiver's breasts and the receiver can reach back to manually stimulate the giver. As this position can be restrictive for the giver, negotiate a signal, such as two sharp taps on the top of the receiver's leg, so the giver can communicate that they need to make immediate adjustments.

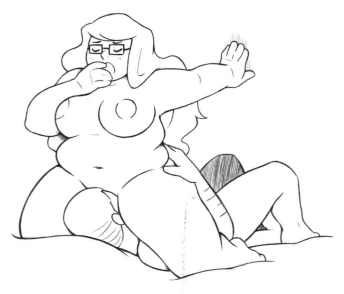

Myth: Crushing

Fat people do not crush their partners during sex. No doubt, sex is inelegant at best, and not just for people of size. We *all* have sex-related mishaps or injuries. They are most often due to the inevitable clumsiness of sex. No one seems to think of a petite woman being in harm's way when her boyfriend is more than three times her weight. Basketball legend Shaquille O'Neal is over seven

7 feet (2 m) tall and 320 pounds (145 kg) and dated a woman for years who was 5 feet, 4 inches (1.5 m) and 100 pounds (45 kg). Guess what? She's alive and well. Don't worry that you will crush your partner or that your partner will crush you. Simply make sure you and your partner are comfortable, and you'll have nothing to worry about.

> Fat people who love themselves scare the shit out of people who don't love themselves. Even fat people who are trying to love themselves scare the shit out of people who can't do the same. We force people to have to look at why they hate their bodies because we are "supposed" to hate ours and we don't. And sometimes they have no idea what to do with that, so they act like assholes.
>
> **Tigress Osborn**

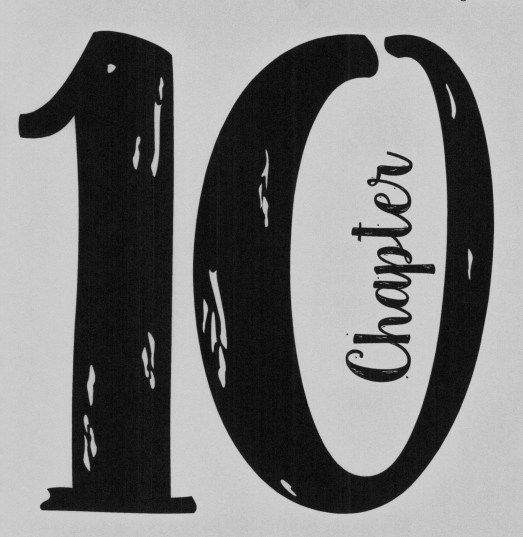

Chapter

10

Other Ways
TO GET IT ON

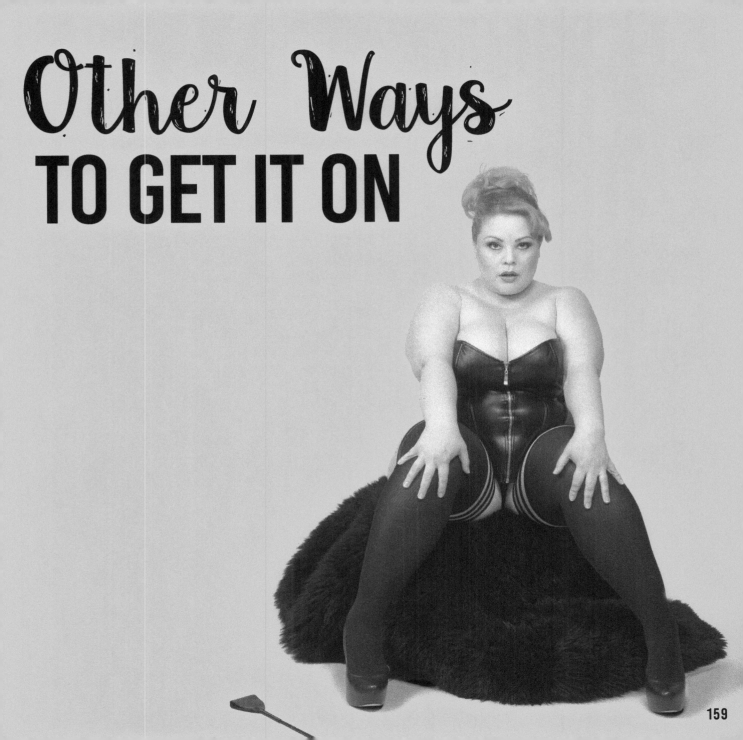

There's a time and a place for everything, and that's especially true when it comes to sex.

Sex in different positions is what this book is all about, but what about the sexual endeavors that don't fit into any of the former categories? Hollywood is always romanticizing what sudden sex looks like on a stairwell, in a car, or even just sex in the water. Sometimes, as curvy gals we can think that that kind of spontaneity isn't for us because some of us need to think about pillow support, or moving tummies to the side, or maybe that we won't fit or get stuck, or can't lean on our knees or hands too long. Well, that's just plain untrue. In this chapter, not only will I show you how to have sex in some of the most popular, unconventional spaces, but I'll also introduce you to some you may not have thought of. The following seventeen positions are a fun grab bag of sex play in and out of the bedroom.

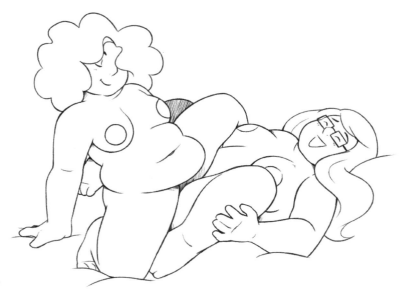

There's the Rub

Frottage has a few definitions that differ in intent and practice, but for the purposes of this book, it is the practice of rubbing your genitals against something or someone for sexual pleasure, without penetration. Some people like rubbing against inanimate objects, such as sofa arms, mattresses, pillows, etc. Still others enjoy the feeling of rubbing up against the skin of their partner. Because curvy gals can have more flesh to worship, this maneuver can be very satisfying for those that love frottage. Don't be shy to use all that you have to your advantage! Offering up some tummy folds or ample butt cheeks to rub his penis between, or inviting him to thrust between thighs or feet might just blow your partner's mind.

Here are some hot frottage ideas:

- The receiver straddles the giver's thigh and grinds against it to stimulate the vulva.
- The receiver lies on her back with a pillow supporting her hips. The giver kneels between her legs and rubs his erect penis or a dildo up and down against the vulva and clitoris.
- The giver lies on his back while the receiver straddles him and rubs her vulva and clitoris against his erect penis.

Stringing the Pearls

This activity is a boob lover's dream, especially because curvy gals have more cushion for the pushin'. Stringing the Pearls (which you might know as a Pearl Necklace) is perfect for fulfilling your penis-wielding paramour's fantasy. The receiver lies on her back with her legs flat on the bed or her knees up and feet flat on the bed. The giver faces the receiver and straddles her torso right below her chest. The receiver holds her breasts together while the giver thrusts his penis in between them, ultimately ejaculating on the receiver's chest and neck. I suggest using lube for this task to avoid chafing on either partner.

"When you've got a partner you're comfortable with, exploring can be so much fun! Go on a scavenger hunt for 'yesses.' See how many things you and your partner can find that please each other. There's no losing that game!"

JoEllen Notte, writer, speaker, and researcher

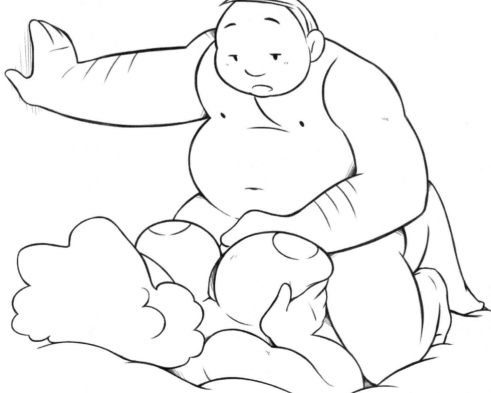

Mutual Masturbation

Mutual masturbation can be a terrific precursor to intercourse, or it can be a main event all on its own. I'm a big proponent of mutual masturbation for couples looking to reestablish intimacy in their relationship, or new couples who want to learn how their partner likes to be touched. Masturbating each other, or in front of each other, can build anticipation and be part of foreplay. There's so much room to explore. Mutual masturbation can involve any of the following scenarios:

- Each partner masturbating simultaneously while watching each another.
- Each partner manually stimulating the other.
- Either partner watching the other masturbate (which is a great way to see how your partner touches themselves and what feels good to them).

"Curves are like road maps. There is always a new and exciting turn ahead to discover. What fun would it be just going from point A to point B? You would miss all the nuances."

**Mistress Simone,
sex columnist and dominatrix**

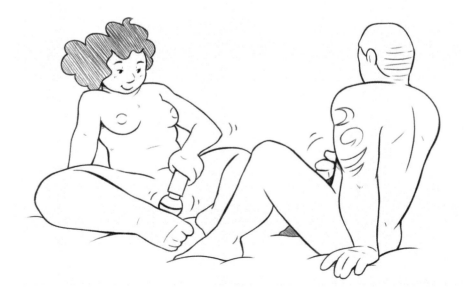

Curvy Strap-On Sex

The giver dons a harness and the dildo of choice (see page 38 for suggestions) while the receiver chooses a comfortable position. From here, partners can engage in any penetrative sexual position. Try this: The receiver lies back on the bed, with her butt at the edge, and lifts one leg in the air while the other dangles off the bed. The giver stands between her legs, holds the upward-pointing leg to her chest, and enters with the strap-on dildo.

Elle's Big Girl Move

Another option for those that don't want to wear a conventional harness is the thigh harness. A thigh harness is a stretchy piece of fabric with a Velcro closure (kind of like an athletic knee support). In the center of the thigh harness is a prefabricated slot to hold your dildo. The giver straps and fastens the harness around her thigh so it's nice and secure but not too tight. The giver can then lie down on the bed or sit up in a chair, and the receiver can straddle the thigh and bring herself down on the dildo. The thigh harness is terrific if the receiver wants to control the action by bobbing up and down on the dildo. Then again, the giver can also move her thigh to provide motion. Experiment and see what's best for you!

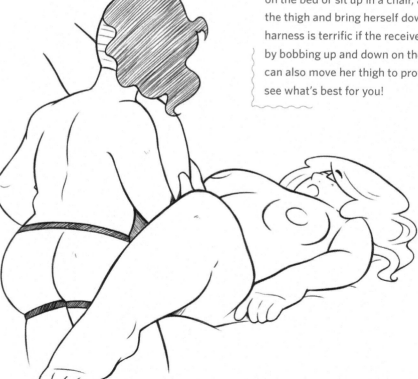

Up the Stairs

Step up and take sex to the next level. The receiver sits at the top step, legs spread and feet firmly planted on whichever step is most comfortable. The receiver then lies back on the landing and welcomes the giver to kneel in between her thighs and line up his penis with her genitals (or anus) and plow away. Consider putting a towel down, especially if the stairs aren't carpeted, to catch any lube spills. Should the stairs have a railing, use that to your advantage and hold on for stability and leverage.

"Lie in bed (blindfold optional). Set the timer for one or two minutes, and have your partner kiss the parts of you that they find stunning while they tell you why they think you are sexy. You don't get to respond until the timer goes off. It's so easy to brush away compliments, but when you *have* to listen without negating or even responding, it's easier to let those positive statements soak in a little more."

Shanna Katz, M.Ed., ACS, ShannaKatz.com

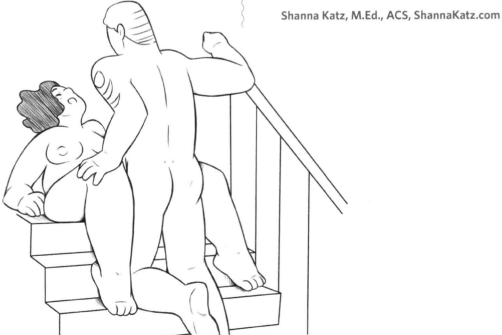

The Sacred Yoni Massage (Vulva Massage)

Yoni (or vulva) massage is a sensual practice where orgasm is not the goal, but receiving and accepting pleasure without reciprocation is. The intent of yoni massage is to honor the receiver and to deepen the trust and intimacy between herself and the giver. Also it feels great! The receiver reclines comfortably, with her legs spread wide, knees bent, and feet on the bed. The giver positions himself between the receiver's legs, either kneeling or cross-legged. The giver uses coconut oil (even silicone lubricant will do) to start the ritual by massaging the receiver's hips, legs, thighs, and belly. He might graze or kiss the area around the vulva, like the mons, or the crevice between the outer labia and the thigh, before finally arriving at the vulva. The giver should take time to gently explore by lightly massaging the labial folds between the fingers and trying different tactile sensations like grazing, light tapping, and lengthwise strokes, always keeping attention on the receiver's responses for guidance. Explore like this on the clitoris as well, but stay focused. Feeling pleasure without the pressure of having an orgasm is the goal . . . but if she has one, that works, too!

"Sometimes I watch smaller bodies getting thrown around, lifted up against walls and doors, and shifted effortlessly in porn, and I feel like I'm missing out. I love it when a partner is able to move and manipulate my body with a combination of strength and accoutrements. The Sport-sheets Door Jam Sex Sling can hold up to 300 pounds (136 kg) and gives me that antigravity feeling that I've been craving. I can completely relax without trying to hold up my body to make myself lighter. "

Ashley Manta, sexuality educator

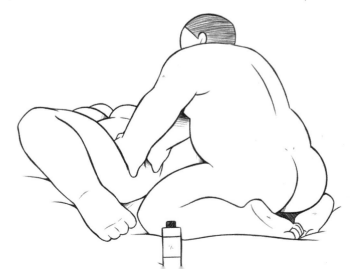

Fooling Around in the Pool

Being in the water renders us weightless, allowing folds and flesh to easily float out of the way. But before you take the plunge, grab some silicone lubricant (it's not water soluble!) and apply it to the genitals. You only need a little to start some underwater stroking. In a public pool or Jacuzzi? You can still get sexy without getting arrested. Use this opportunity to start the teasing, and then blow your lifeguard's . . . whistle because it's everybody out of the pool!

Rub-A-Dub-Dub

If you're really craving some tub lovin', cowboy-style is your best bet. The giver sits in the tub, and the receiver straddles him. Her bent knees rest atop his thighs against the sides of the tub. Motion should be slow and deep to keep water from splashing outside the tub. She can get close to him by pressing her chest against his (he can wrap his arms around her, if he likes) and raising and lowering her hips for less water disturbance. Alternatively, she can steady herself by placing her hands on the wall behind him or on the sides of the tub.

Elle's Big Girl Move

It may be counterintuitive, but water actually isn't a natural lubricant. In fact, it will dry up any wetness you're producing naturally. Shower or bathtub sex really requires silicone lube because it can stand up to water, and a little goes a long way. Be warned that silicone lube is *very* slick, which makes the bottom of the shower or tub dangerous. My suggestion? Slather a little silicone-based lube on the penis or dildo *before* jumping in the shower, or get yourself something called a *lube shooter*. Lube shooters are small plastic cylinders with a plunger. Fill it up with lube and, when you're ready to get down, just insert the shooter into the vagina (or anus) and use the plunger to deposit the lube inside you. Step carefully when you're done, as some lube will probably leak out and be underfoot. You can also use suction cup handles and foot rests to help keep you steady and upright during your special shower time.

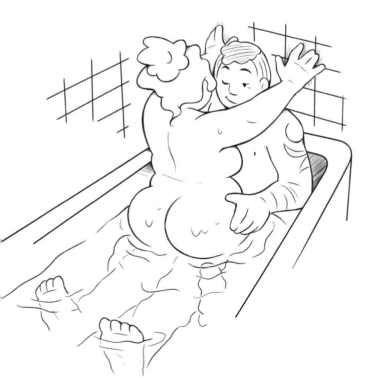

Sex in the Shower

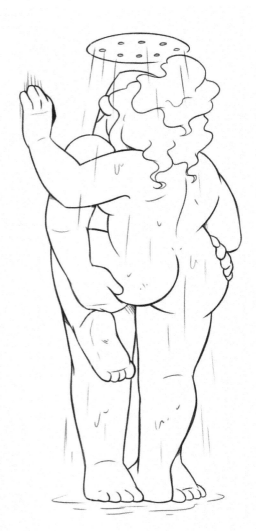

Sex in the shower is one of those things that, as a curvy gal, I never felt comfortable doing until recently. After I got over what I thought I looked like nude and wet with mascara running down my face, I found that working out a position ahead of time in which I felt physically stable and sexy was the key to success. Stand facing each other in the shower. Both partners embrace, arms wrapped around each other. The receiver should wrap a leg around the giver's thigh, hips, or waist (whichever is most comfortable). The giver then places a hand under the receiver's lifted thigh to help them both stay steady, and enters. If tummies are making entry challenging, there's nothing in the rulebook* that says either one of you can't lift up a tummy or two in order to get going. Once penetration ensues, the giver and receiver can use free hands to stimulate the clit, passionately grab a fistful of hair or slap a butt cheek. Just remember to be careful not to slip, especially if you're using a bit of silicone lube in your play. By the time you're done with this shower, you'll need another one!

*I jest. There is no rulebook.

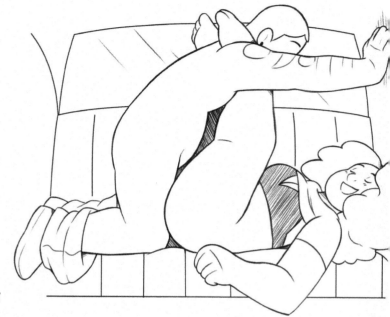

Curvy Car Missionary

I've always had a thing for sex in cars, and apparently I'm not alone. Some studies suggest that not only is sex in a car one of the top fantasies women have, but that 50% of us have tried it. If you haven't but want to, you can start with simple missionary. The receiver lies across the backseat and brings her knees in toward her chest. The giver kneels with his knees close to the receiver's butt and supports her calves on his shoulders as he enters. The receiver has the option to press her feet against the roof of the car and use her legs for thrusting leverage, or spreading her legs wider and anchoring her feet wherever is most comfortable.

Elle's Big Girl Move

As a big girl myself, I love this classic position. In Curvy Car Missionary, woman with a larger stomach can manually pull back her tummy as her lover begins to enter her. Her thighs can keep her tummy in place, holding the flesh away from the action for easier entry. Because the hips are naturally lifted higher in this position, your partner will find he has more room to move and will be able to position his body to get at just the right angle for his pleasure—and yours. This can also be wonderful for G-spot stimulation, especially if your lover has a curve to his penis or is using a dildo with a curve. Now get at it and steam up some windows!

Curvy Car Cowgirl

Yee haw! If possible, pull the front seats forward and push the backs down toward the windshield. The giver sits in the center of the backseat with his knees bent, legs extended, and feet resting on the backs of the front seats, or he can leave his feet on the floor. The receiver faces the giver, straddles him, and slides down onto the penis. The receiver can rest her hands on the top of the backseat for support while bouncing on the penis or dildo. The giver's hands are free to lift the stomach and massage the clitoris, spread the butt cheeks or labial folds, massage the breasts, or simply hold the receiver close while thrusting.

Curvy Car Reverse Cowgirl

If possible, pull the front seats forward and push the backs down toward the windshield. The giver sits in the center of the backseat with his legs extended, knees bent, and feet resting on the backs of the front seats, or he can leave his feet on the floor. The receiver faces the front of the car, straddles the giver, and slides down onto the penis. The receiver can keep her feet on the floor of the car or her shins on the backseat on either side of her partner. The receiver can press her hands to the ceiling of the car, or lean all the way forward and rest her hands on the back of the front seats to maintain balance and get leverage for grinding. Alternatively, she can lie forward against the giver's legs, allowing him to thrust. From there, the giver is also free to spread the receiver's butt cheeks, or lift his own tummy for ease of penetration or to stimulate the anus.

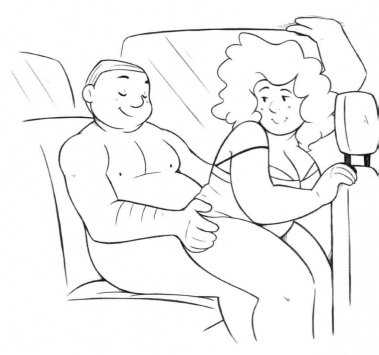

Curvy Car Doggy Style

The receiver gets on her hands and knees on the backseat, facing one of the side windows. The giver gets behind her, with one knee on the car seat between the receiver's legs and the other foot on the floor of the car, then leans forward and enters. The giver's hands may grip the receiver's hips for greater thrusting leverage, spread her butt cheeks and/or thighs for easier access or for deeper penetration, or massage her breasts and vulva.

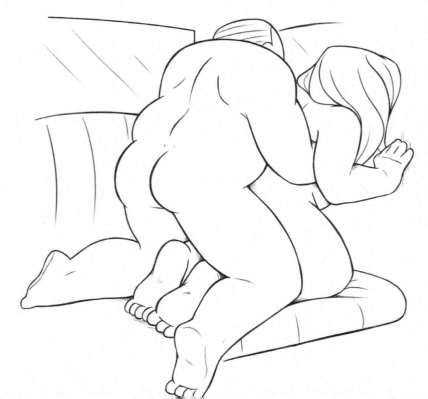

Curvy Car Fellatio

The classic "road head" position involves the receiver (this time, the man) sitting in the driver's seat (in a parked car) and the giver in the passenger seat. The giver remains seated and leans over to fellate the receiver. You can see why this may not be safe while driving! The challenge here can be the giver's breasts and/or the "driver's" larger belly. The receiver will have to adjust her breasts to get comfortable, or ask the receiver to help keep them out of the way. If the receiver's belly obstructs access, he can try reclining the seat or holding back the belly, whichever is easiest. This works nicely for a good hand job, as well.

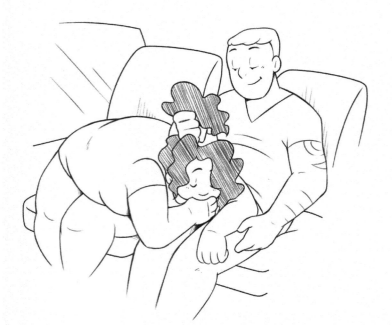

Elle's Big Girl Move

Getting (and giving) a blow-job in a car is a part of exhibitionistic, voyeuristic, role-play and otherwise erotic fantasies for a lot of people. It can be very exciting—and safe, as long as the car isn't being operated by one of you at the same time. Have a drive-in movie theatre where you live? Taking a road trip? Map out where there might be some service roads on the way that could be private enough for a roadside rendezvous. If the coast is clear, surprise your lover when you unexpectedly turn onto the secluded spot and begin to go for the jewels. Pick your partner up from work one day wearing something you feel sexy in, and drive him into a secluded area for some front-seat fun. Or for a less risky method, wait for your partner in the garage when he's on the way home, or be in the car waiting in the morning before he leaves, and seduce him right then and there. It really doesn't matter what the circumstances are—blowing your partner in a car is sexy, but add a new location, scenario, or fantasy and you have a recipe for a mind-blowing good time.

Curvy Car Cunnilingus

The receiver lies down on her back in the backseat, with her legs spread and extended. Depending on the car and the footwear, one of the receiver's feet can rest on the ceiling or front seat, and the other can rest on the headrest of the backseat or the back window. The giver kneels on the floor of the backseat and leans in to service the receiver, or sits or kneels on the backseat in front of the receiver and leans over to dine.

Elle's Big Girl Move

When we think of car sex, we probably conjure up images of being in a convertible, parked on a hill overlooking city lights, and when things get hot and heavy, the couple disappears into the comfort of the car seat. In real life, comfortable car sex benefits from some forethought and preparation. For instance, if you have leather seats in your car, you'll thank me for suggesting that you carry a throw or a large towel in the car. When hot, naked, sweaty body parts come in contact with leather or vinyl, it can get slippery or sticky. Just try not to wince or scream in pain when you rip your sweaty bum from the leather seat and feel the searing "burn." Place that towel or blanket underneath and/or behind you. Your skin will thank you.

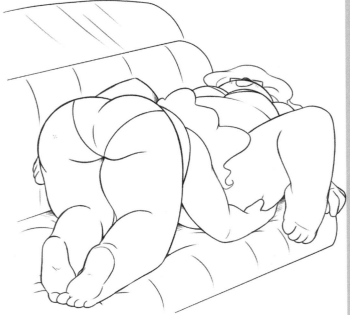

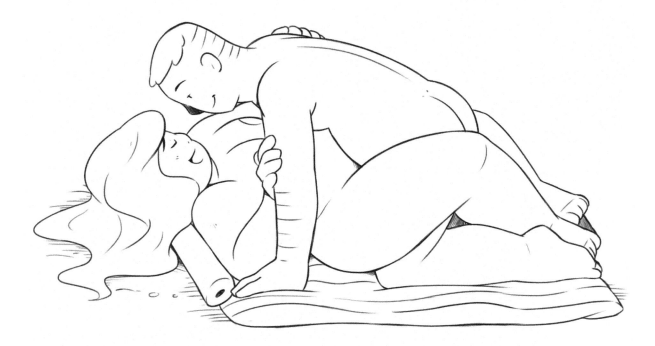

The Great Outdoors

Get ready for "in-tents" sexual fun! Who says sex in the great outdoors means roughing it? With a little planning, you can still have all the comfortable camping sex your heart desires. If you enjoy pillows and props at home for comfy sex, the camping versions are inexpensive to create, and you might already own some of what's needed. In the great outdoors, inflatables are your best friend. Pool toys like floats and water wings—even pool noodles—are surprisingly effective for propping up heads and hips, and inflatable rafts are great for cushioning over a pine-needly ground, log, or boulder. Here is my favorite fix: Stuff a sleeping bag with a few pool noodles, lengthwise. Zip up the sleeping bag and use it to prop up the receiver's hips, just like you would use pillows at home. Use a couple of rectangular pool rafts to cushion your tushy on a hard ground, and voilà, you have comfortable, easy-access sex just by MacGyvering some supplies you're probably packing anyway.

Curvy Girl on the Hood

Feeling exhibitionistic? Have a private garage? Then sex on the hood of the car can be scorching hot! For larger or less nimble receivers, choosing a car that is lower to the ground is your best bet here. For this advanced position, the receiver can lie on her back, with her tush right at the edge of the front of the hood. The giver can hold on to her ankles, place them on his shoulders, or just keep them in the air and spread 'em for some motorway missionary. Alternatively, the receiver can bend at the waist and support herself by planting her hands on the hood of the car for some driveway doggie style, or even lie back and enjoy a little oral al fresco while placing one foot on the hood and letting the other one dangle so the giver can ravish your nether-regions while you enjoy a view of the night sky—or the ceiling of your garage.

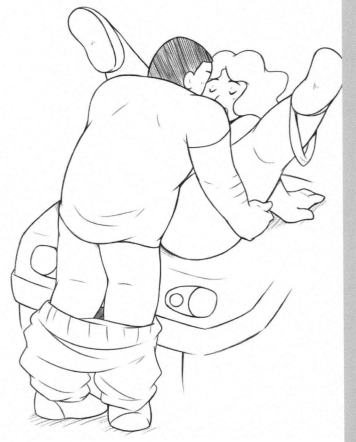

Curvy Resources

Curvy Girl Reading

Bacon, Linda. *Health at Every Size: The Surprising Truth about Your Weight*. Dallas, TX: BenBella, 2008.

Baker, Jes. *Things No One Will Tell Fat Girls: A Handbook for Unapologetic Living*. Berkeley, CA: Seal Press, 2015.

Batts, Carlos. *Fat Girl*. Los Angeles, CA: Rare Bird, 2013.

Blank, Hanne. *Big Big Love: A Sourcebook on Sex for People of Size and Those Who Love Them*. Emeryville, CA: Greenery press, 2000.

Blank, Hanne. *The Unapologetic Fat Girl's Guide to Exercise and Other Incendiary Acts*. Berkeley, CA: Ten Speed Press, 2012.

Boston Women's Health Collective. *Our Bodies, Ourselves: A New Edition for a New Era*. New York, NY: Touchstone, 2005.

Brach, Tara. *Radical Acceptance: Embracing Your Life with the Heart of a Buddha*. New York, NY: Bantam Dell, 2003.

Brown, Brené. *Daring Greatly: How the Courage to Be Vulnerable Transforms the Way We Live, Love, Parent, and Lead*. New York, NY: Gotham, 2012.

Brown, Brené. *I Thought It Was Just Me (but It Isn't): Telling the Truth about Perfectionism, Inadequacy, and Power*. New York, NY: Gotham, 2008.

Brown, Brené. *The Gifts of Imperfection: Let Go of Who You Think You're Supposed to Be and Embrace Who You Are*. Center City, MN: Hazelden; 1 edition, 2010.

Brown, Harriet. *Body of Truth: How Science, History, and Culture Drive Our Obsession with Weight--and What We Can Do about It*. Boston, MA: Da Capo Press; reprint edition, 2016.

Brumfitt, Taryn. *Embrace: My Story from Body Loather to Body Lover. Paperback*. New Holland, Australia: New Holland Publishers, 2015.

Bussel, Rachel Kramer. *Curvy Girls: Erotica for Women*. Berkeley, CA: Seal Press, 2012.

Cohen, Alan. *Why Your Life Sucks: And What You Can Do about It*. San Diego, CA: Jodere Group, 2002.

Cole-Whittaker, Terry. *What You Think of Me Is None of My Business*. New York, NY: Jove, 1988.

Fleming, Lauren Marie. *Bawdy Love: 10 Steps to Profoundly Loving Your Body*. 1st ed. Eugene, OR: Bordista Media, 2015 Print.

Friedman, Jaclyn, and Jessica Valenti. *Yes Means Yes!: Visions of Female Sexual Power & a World without Rape*. Berkeley, CA: Seal Press, 2008.

Gibbons, Brittany. *Fat Girl Walking: Sex, Food, Love, and Being Comfortable in Your Skin--Every Inch of It*. New York, NY: Dey Street Books; reprint edition,, 2015.

Haines, Staci. *The Survivor's Guide to Sex: How to Have an Empowered Sex Life After Child Sexual Abuse*. San Francisco, CA: Cleis Press, 1999.

Harding, Kate, and Marianne Kirby. *Lessons from the Fat-o-sphere: Quit Dieting and Declare a Truce with Your Body*. New York, NY: Perigee Book, 2009.

Hay, Louise L. *Love Your Body: A Positive Affirmation Guide for Loving and Appreciating Your Body*. London: Hay House, 1989.

Kaufman, Miriam. *The Ultimate Guide to Sex and Disability: For All of Us Who Live with Disabilities, Chronic Pain, and Illness*. San Francisco, CA: Cleis Press, 2007.

Kotkin, Alex, *#NSFW Totally Curvy Coloring Book* - Edited by Lady Cheeky, New York, NY: SheVibe Studios, 2017.

Kotkin, Alex, *#NSFW Totally Naughty Coloring Book* - Edited by Lady Cheeky, New York, NY: SheVibe Studios, 2016.

Madsen, Pamela. *Shameless: How I Ditched the Diet, Got Naked, Found True Pleasure ... and Somehow Got Home in Time to Cook Dinner*. Emmaus, PA: Rodale, 2011.

Miller, Kelsey. *Big Girl: How I Gave up Dieting and Got a Life*. New York, NY: Grand Central Publishing, 2016.

Molinary, Rosie. *Beautiful You: A Daily Guide to Radical Self-acceptance*. Berkeley, CA: Seal Press, 2010.

Molinary, Rosie. *Hijas Americanas: Beauty, Body Image, and Growing Up Latina*. Berkeley, CA: Seal Press; annotated edition, 2007.

Nimoy, Leonard. *The Full Body Project*. Brooklyn, NY: Five Ties, 2007.

Sicero, Jen. *You Are a Badass: How to Stop Doubting Your Greatness and Start Living an Awesome Life*. Philadelphia, PA: Running Press; 1 edition. 2013.

Tovar, Virgie. *Hot & Heavy: Fierce Fat Girls on Life, Love & Fashion*. Berkeley, CA: Seal Press, 2012.

Valenti, Jessica. *Sex Object: A Memoir*. New York, NY: Dey Street Books, 2016.

Wann, Marilyn. *Fat! So?: Because You Don't Have to Apologize for Your Size!* Berkeley, CA: Ten Speed Press, 1998.

Weinstein, Rebecca Jane. *Fat Sex: The Naked Truth*. N.p.: Createspace Independent Pub., 2012.

West, Lindy. *Shrill: Notes from a Loud Woman*. New York, NY: Hachette Books, 2016.

Williamson, Marianne. *A Woman's Worth*. New York, NY: Random House, 1993.

Wolf, Naomi. *The Beauty Myth: How Images of Beauty Are Used against Women*. New York, NY: W. Morrow, 1991.

Wolf, Naomi. *Vagina: A New Biography*. New York, NY: Ecco, 2012.

Ziel, Cornelia Van Der, and Jacqueline Tourville. *Big, Beautiful & Pregnant*. New York, NY: Marlowe & Company, 2006.

Zilbergeld, B. *The New Male Sexuality: The Truth About Men, Sex, and Pleasure*. New York, NY: Bantam, 1999.

Sex & Kink Education & How To

Block, Jenny. *O Wow: Discovering Your Ultimate Orgasm*. San Francisco, CA: Cleis Press, 2015.

Carrellas, Barbara. *Ecstasy Is Necessary: A Practical Guide*. Carlsbad, CA: Hay House, 2012.

Carrellas, Barbara. *Urban Tantra: Sacred Sex for the Twenty-first Century*. Berkeley, CA: Celestial Arts, 2007.

Corinna, Heather. *S.E.X., Second Edition: The All-You-Need-To-Know Sexuality Guide to Get You Through Your Teens and Twenties*. 2nd ed. Boston, MA: Da Capo Lifelong, 2016.

Daedone, Nicole. *Slow Sex: The Art and Craft of the Female Orgasm*. New York, NY: Grand Central Life & Style, 2011.

Dodson, Betty. *Sex for One: The Joy of Selfloving*. New York, NY: Crown Trade Paperbacks, 1996.

DooLittle, Ducky. *Sex with the Lights On: 200 Illuminating Sex Questions Answered*. New York, NY: Carroll & Graf, 2006.

Friedman, Jaclyn. *What You Really Really Want: The Smart Girl's Shame-free Guide to Sex and Safety*. Berkeley, CA: Seal Press, 2011.

Glickman, Charlie, and Aislinn Emirzian. *The Ultimate Guide to Prostate Pleasure: Erotic Exploration for Men and Their Partners*. Berkeley, CA: Cleis Press, 2013.

Hartley, Nina, and I. S. Levine. *Nina Hartley's Guide to Total Sex*. New York, NY: Avery, 2006.

Hasler, Nikol, and Michael Capozzola. *Sex: An Uncensored Introduction*. San Francisco, CA: Zest, 2015.

Herbenick, Debby, and Vanessa Schick. *Read My Lips: A Complete Guide to the Vagina and Vulva*. Lanham: Washington, DC: Rowman & Littlefield, 2011.

Herbenick, Debby. *Because It Feels Good: A Woman's Guide to Sexual Pleasure and Satisfaction*. Emmaus, PA: Rodale, 2009.

Horn, Tina. *Sexting: The Grownup's Little Book of Sex Tips for Getting Dirty Digitally*. Beverly, MA: Quiver, 2016.

Jaiya. *Sex Positions You Never Thought Possible: The Creators of the Liberator Wedge Show You the Secrets of the Angles and Inclinations for the Deepest, Most Orgasmic Sex Ever*. Beverly, MA: Quiver, 2012.

Joannides, Paul, and Dærick Gross. *Guide to Getting It On: A Book about the Wonders of Sex*. Waldport, OR: Goofy Foot: 2012.

Katz, Shanna. *Lesbian Sex Positions: 100 Passionate Positions from Intimate and Sensual to Wild and Naughty*. Berkeley, CA: Amorata, 2014.

Kaufman, Miriam, Cory Silverberg, and Fran Odette. *The Ultimate Guide to Sex and Disability: For All of Us Who Live with Disabilities, Chronic Pain, and Illness*. San Francisco, CA: Cleis Press, 2003.

Kerner, Ian. *She Comes First: The Thinking Man's Guide to Pleasuring a Woman*. New York, NY: Regan, 2004.

Moon, Allison, and Kate Diamond. *Girl Sex 101*. Nanaimo, British Columbia: Lunatic Ink, 2015.

Murray, Rowena A. *For Foxes' Sake: Everything a Fox Needs to Know about Sex*. Print ed. N.p.: Amazon Digital Services, 2016.

Nagoski, Emily. *Come as You Are: The Surprising New Science That Will Transform Your Sex Life*. New York, NY: Simon & Schuster, 2015.

Price, Joan. *Naked at Our Age: Talking out Loud about Senior Sex*. Berkeley, CA: Seal Press, 2011.

Taormino, Tristan. *The Secrets of Great G-spot Orgasms and Female Ejaculation: The Best Positions and Latest Techniques for Creating Powerful, Long-lasting Full-body Orgasms*. Beverly, MA: Quiver, 2011.

Taormino, Tristan. *The Ultimate Guide to Anal Sex for Women*. San Francisco, CA: Cleis Press, 1998.

Taormino, Tristan. *The Ultimate Guide to Kink: BDSM, Role Play and the Erotic Edge*. Berkeley, CA: Cleis Press, 2012.

Waxman, Jamye, Emily Morse, and Benjamin Wachenje. *Hot Sex: Over 200 Things You Can Try Tonight*. San Francisco, CA: Weldon Owen, 2011.

Waxman, Jamye. *Getting Off: A Woman's Guide to Masturbation*. Emeryville, CA: Seal Press, 2007.

Winston, Sheri. *Women's Anatomy of Arousal: Secret Maps to Buried Pleasure*. Kingston, NY: Mango Garden, 2010.

Gender

Bornstein, Kate, and S. Bear Bergman. *Gender Outlaws: The next Generation*. Berkeley, CA: Seal Press; reprint edition, 2010.

Bornstein, Kate. *A Queer and Pleasant Danger: The True Story of a Nice Jewish Boy Who Joins the Church of Scientology, and Leaves Twelve Years Later to Become the Lovely Lady She Is Today*. Boston, MA: Beacon, 2013.

Bornstein, Kate. *Gender Outlaw: On Men, Women, and the Rest of Us*. New York, NY: Routledge, 1994.

Bornstein, Kate. *My New Gender Workbook: A Step-by-step Guide to Achieving World Peace through Gender Anarchy and Sex Positivity*. New York, NY: Routledge, 2013.

Boylan, Jennifer Finney. *She's Not There: A Life in Two Genders*. New York, NY: Crown Publishing Group, 2003.

Feinberg, Leslie. *Transgender Warriors: Making History from Joan of Arc to RuPaul*. Boston, MA: Beacon, 1996.

Girshick, Lori B. *Transgender Voices: Beyond Women and Men*. Hanover: Lebanon, NH: U of New England, 2008.

Mock, Janet. *Redefining Realness: My Path to Womanhood, Identity, Love & so Much More*. New York, NY: Atria Books; reprint edition, 2014.

Serano, Julia. *Whipping Girl: A Transsexual Woman on Sexism and the Scapegoating of Femininity*. Berkeley, CA: Seal Press, 2016.

Sexuality, Sensuality & Relationships

Bechdel, Alison. *Fun Home: A Family Tragicomic*. Boston, MA: Houghton Mifflin, 2006.

Chalker, Rebecca. *The Clitoral Truth*. New York, NY: Seven Stories Press, 2000.

Donaghue, Chris. *Sex outside the Lines: Authentic Sexuality in a Sexually Dysfunctional Culture*. Dallas, TX: BenBella Books, 2015.

Goddard, Amy Jo. *Woman on Fire: 9 Elements to Wake up Your Erotic Energy, Personal Power, and Sexual Intelligence*. New York, NY: Avery, 2015.

Hills, Rachel. *The Sex Myth: The Gap between Our Fantasies and Reality*. New York, NY: Simon & Schuster, 2015.

Michaels, Mark A., and Patricia Johnson. *Designer Relationships: A Guide to Happy Monogamy, Positive Polyamory, and Optimistic Open Relationships*. Berkeley, CA: Cleis Press, 2015.

Michaels, Mark A., and Patricia Johnson. *Partners in Passion*. Berkeley, CA: Cleis Press, 2014.

Perel, Esther. *Mating in Captivity: Unlocking Erotic Intelligence*. New York, NY: Harper, 2007.

Taormino, Tristan. *Opening Up: A Guide to Creating and Sustaining Open Relationships*. San Francisco, CA: Cleis Press, 2008.

Erotica Favorites

Blank, Hanne. *Zaftig: Well Rounded Erotica*. San Francisco, CA: Cleis Press, 2001.

Blue, Violet. *Best of Best Women's Erotica 2*. San Francisco, CA: Cleis Press, 2010.

Bussel, Rachel Kramer. *Curvy Girls: Erotica for Women*. Berkeley, CA: Seal Press, 2012.

Bussel, Rachel Kramer, and Barbara Carrellas. *The Big Book of Orgasms: 69 Sexy Stories*. Berkeley, CA: Cleis Press, 2013.

Caraway, Rose. *The Sexy Librarian's Big Book of Erotica*. New York, NY: Simon & Schuster, 2014.

Nin, Anais. *Delta of Venus. Erotica by Anais Nin*. London: Allen, 1978. P.

Réage, Pauline, *The Story of O*. New York, NY: Ballantine Books, 2013.

Roquelaure, A. N., Rice, Anne. The Sleeping Beauty Novels: *The Claiming of Sleeping Beauty / Beauty's Release / Beauty's Punishment 1st* (first): St, Lawrence, MA: Plume Printing, 1999.

Taormino, Tristan, and Ali Liebegott. *When She Was Good: Best Lesbian Erotica*. Berkeley, CA: Cleis Press, 2014.

Taormino, Tristan. *Take Me There: Trans and Genderqueer Erotica*. Berkeley, CA: Cleis Press, 2011.

Wright, Kristina. *Best Erotic Romance of the Year*. Berkeley, CA: Cleis press, 2015.

Plus Sized Lingerie Websites

About Curves, www.aboutcurves.com

Additionelle, www.additionelle.com

Adore Me, www.adoreme.com

Ashley Stewart, www.ashleystewart.com

Bare Necessities, www.barenecessities.com

Big Gals Lingerie, www.biggalslingerie.com

Bigger Bras, www.biggerbras.com

Bits of Lace, www.bitsoflace.com

Breast Nest, www.breastnest.com

Fig Leaves, www.figleaves.com

Her Room, www.herroom.com

Hips and Curves, www.hipsandcurves.com

Lace, www.lace.com

Lane Bryant, www.lanebryant.com

Les Love Boat, www.lesloveboat.com

Leslee Valise, www.leeleesvalise.com

Soma, www.soma.com

Torrid, www.torrid.com

Underworks, www.underworks.com

Curvy Girl-Approved Toys & Products for Curvy Bodies

Dildos

Clone-A-Willy, www.cloneawilly.com

Fun Factory, www.funfactory.com
SHARE

New York Toy Collective, www.newyorktoycollective.com
Mason

Njoy, www.njoytoys.com
Fun Wand and Pure Wand

Good Vibrations, www.goodvibrations.com
PleasureWorks Admiral

Tantus, www.tauntusinc.com
Echo Handle, Feeldoe, G-Force, and Goddess Handle

Harnesses

Aslan Leather, www.aslanleather.com
Minx Upgrade, Pleasure Harness

The Pleasure Chest, www.thepleasurechest.com
Harness Extender Strap

SpareParts, www.myspare.com
Bella, Joque, Sasha, and Tomboi

Spartacus, www.shopspartacus.com
Leather Ulti-Mate Harness

SportSheets, www.sportsheets.com
Divine Diva Plus Sized Strap-On Harness

Tantus, www.tantusinc.com
Vibrating Velvet Harness

Packers/Gender Identity

Good Vibrations, www.goodvibrations.com
Pleasure Works Sailor Soft Pack

New York Toy Collective, www.newyorktoycollective.com
Archer (circumcised) and Pierre (uncircumcised) silicone packers

The Pleasure Chest, www.thepleasurechest.com
BodyPerks Nipple Enhancers and Transform Full Triangle Breast Forms

Props & Accessories

SheVibe, www.shevibe.com
Pipedream Fetish Fantasy Door Swing

Liberator, www.liberator.com
Ramp, Slingshot, and Wedge

Sportsheets, www.sportsheets.com
Door Jam Sex Sling, Penetration Station, Plus Size Doggy Strap, and Super Sex Sling

Sybian, www.sybian.com

In the Shower

Amazon.com or medical supply sites
Suction handles, bars, and footrests

Sportsheets, www.sportsheets.com
Dual Locking Suction Handle, Single Locking Suction Footrest, Single Locking Suction Handle, and Suction Hand Cuffs

Lube

Water-based

Sliquid, www.sliquid.com
Naturals and Organics Intimate Lubricants

Pjur, www.pjur.com

Please, www.goodvibrations.com
Liquid, cream, or gel

Flavored (water-based)

Sliquid, www.sliquid.com
Swirl

Wicked Sensual Care, www.wickedsensualcare.com

Silicone

Good Vibrations, www.goodvibrations.com
Please Silicone Lubricant

Pjur, www.pjurlove.com

Sliquid, www.sliquid.com
Silver

Uberlube, www.uberlube.com

Hybrid

Ride Bodyworx, www.ridelube.com
Silk Hybrid

Sliquid, www.sliquid.com
Silk

Oil-based (not safe with condoms)

Organic, extra-virgin, fractionated coconut oil, available at any supermarket or health food store

Sex Butter, www.sexbutter.net

Sexual Health Products

Aneros, www.aneros.com
EVI kegel exerciser

FC2 Female Condoms, www.fc2femalecondom.com

Lucky Bloke, www.luckybloke.com
Glyde, Okomoto .004, ONE, Skyn, and Unique condoms, and oral sex dams

The Pleasure Chest, www.thepleasurechest.com
Hot Dam non-latex dental dam

Je Joue Ami, www.jejoue.com
Ami and Ami+ kegel exercisers

Minna Life, www.minnalife.com
kGoal kegel trainer

Vibrators (V) / Pulsators (P) / Wands (W)

Doxy, www.doxymassager.com
Doxy Massager (W)

Eroscillator, www.eroscillator.com
Top Deluxe/Soft Finger Combo (V)

Fun Factory, www.funfactory.com
Amorino (V) and Stronic Eins (P)

JeJoue, www.jejoue.com
G-Kii (V)

SheVibe, www.shevibe.com
Key Comet 2 Vibrating G-Spot Wand (V)

L'Amourose, www.lamourose.com
Prism V (V) and Rosa Rouge (V)

Original Magic Wand, www.magicwandoriginal.com
Magic Wand Original (W)

The Screaming O, www.thescreamingo.com
Fing-O (V), Pop Rabbit (V), Pop Vibe (V), and Spork Multi-use Pleasure Tool (V)

Swan Vibes, www.swanvibes.com
Eternal Swan (V), Mute Swan (V), Swan Curve (V), Swan Wand (W), and Trumpeter Swan (V)

Tantus, www.tantusinc.com
Rumble (and all the attachments) (W)

Vibratex, www.vibratex.com
Joystick (V) and Mystic Wand (W)

We-Vibe, www.wevibe.com
4 Plus (V), Nova (V), Rave (V), Tango (V), and Tango Pleasure Mates Collection (V)

Anal Toys

The Stockroom, www.stockroom.com
Anal hooks

Crystal Delights, www.crystaldelights.com
Crystal Kiss anal plug

SheVibe, www.shevibe.com
Fashionistas Rose Glass Butt Plug

Fun Factory, www.funfactory.com
Bootie butt plug

njoy, www.njoytoys.com
Pure Plugs

OhMiBod, www.ohmibod.com
Lovelife Dare and Lovelife Explore butt plugs

Tantus, www.tantusinc.com
Perfect Plug and ProTouch (prostate)

Vibratex, www.Vibratex.com
Black Pearl (prostate)

Body & Sex Positive Adult Shopping

I suggest checking out the internet's most comprehensive listing of sex positive retailers featuring more than 50 shops spanning the U.S. and Canada: The Redhead Bedhead's Superhero Sex Shop List, www.redheadbedhead.com/superhero-sex-shops

As You Like It, www.asyoulikeitshop.com
A sex toy shop that sells non-toxic, gender inclusive, body positive, sex positive, and environmentally conscious sexual health supplies and toys.

A Woman's Touch, www.sexualityresources.com
Women-owned retail and online store featuring toys, books, videos, safer sex supplies, and education.

Babeland, www.babeland.com
Women-owned retail and online stores featuring toys, books, videos, safer sex supplies, and education.

Center For Sexual Pleasure And Health, www.shopthecsph.org
Sex positive online store featuring toys, books, videos, safer sex supplies, and educational materials.

Dallas Novelty, www.dallasnovelty.com
Sex positive online retailer selling sex toys for all, including people with disabilities.

Early to Bed, www.early2bedshop.com
Women-owned retail and online store featuring toys, books, videos, safer sex supplies, and education.

Good Vibrations, www.goodvibrations.com
Sex positive retail and online stores featuring toys, books, videos, safer sex supplies, education, and on-demand ethical porn.

Lotus Blooms, www.lotusblooms.com
Sex positive retail and online stores featuring toys, books, videos, safer sex supplies, and education. Great selection of plus size corsets.

LuckyBloke, www.luckybloke.com
Only the best condoms, dams, lubes, sent to your home in sampler packs or all one brand. You choose!

Self Serve Toys, www.selfservetoys.com
The best in the southwest! Female-friendly and female-owned adult toy store that also offers terrific classes.

The Pleasure Chest, www.thepleasurechest.com
Sex positive retail and online stores featuring toys, books, videos, safer sex supplies, and education. I have my own educator page on the Pleasure Chest site with my recommendations.

She Bop, www.sheboptheshop.com
Women-owned retail and online store featuring toys, books, videos, safer sex supplies, and education.

SheVibe, www.shevibe.com
You'll find what you need at this fun, colorful, and well-stocked site. Also the creator of the #NSFW Totally Naughty Coloring Books

Smitten Kitten, www.smittenkittenonline.com
Women-owned retail and online store featuring toys, books, videos, safer sex supplies, and education.

Sugar, www.sugartheshop.com
Women-owned retail and online store featuring toys, books, videos, safer sex supplies, and education.

SHAG Brooklyn, www.weloveshag.com
Carefully curated boutique with sexy accouterments, from bath and body products to lingerie and sexy toys for all.

The Stockroom, www.stockroom.com
Fetish wear and accoutrements, including plus-size latex outfits and other fetish wear.

Tool Shed, www.toolshedtoys.com
Women-owned retail and online store featuring toys, books, videos, safer sex supplies, and education.

Venus Envy, www.venusenvy.ca
Sex positive retail and online stores featuring toys, books, videos, safer sex supplies, and education.

Sexual Health & Lifestyle Resources

Abortion Clinics Online, www.abortionclinics.com

About Relationships, sexuality.about.com

American Sexual Health Association, www.ashasexualhealth.org

Centers for Disease Control and Prevention (CDC), www.cdc.gov/sexualhealth

CDC National Prevention Information Network, npin.cdc.gov

Center for Reproductive Rights, www.reproductiverights.org

Get Tested, gettested.cdc.gov

Kink Academy, www.kinkacademy.com

Kinsey Confidential, www.kinseyconfidential.org

Naked at Our Age, www.nakedatourage.com

National Domestic Violence Hotline, www.thehotline.org

Options for Sexual Health, www.optionsforsexualhealth.org

Planned Parenthood, www.plannedparenthood.org

Rape, Abuse, Incest National Network, www.rainn.org

San Francisco Sex Information, www.sfsi.org

Scarleteen, www.scarleteen.com

Society of Janus, www.soj.org

The Center for Sexual Pleasure and Health, www.thecsph.org

Women's Health, www.womenshealth.gov

Woodhull Freedom Foundation, www.woodhullfoundation.org

LGBTQ Sexual Health

Advocates for Youth, www.advocatesforyouth.org

American Institute of Bisexuality, www.bisexual.org

Black Girl Dangerous, www.blackgirldangerous.org

Gay Men's Health Crisis, www.gmhc.org

Gay, Lesbian Straight Education Network, www.glsen.org

Gender Wellness of Los Angeles, www.genwell.org

GLAAD, www.glaad.org

Impact Program, www.impactprogram.org

Intersex Society of North America, www.isna.org

LAMBDA Legal, www.lambdalegal.org

National Center for Lesbian Rights, www.nclrights.org

National Center for Transgender Equality, www.nctequality.org

National LGBT Task Force, www.thetaskforce.org

The A-sexual Visability and Education Network, www.asexuality.org

Educator's Websites Mentioned in This Book

Megan Andelloux, www.ohmegan.com

Buck Angel, www.buckangel.com

Barbara Carrellas, www.barbaracarrellas.com

Cyndi Darnell, www.cyndidarnell.com

Catherine Deveny, www.catherinedeveny.com

Betty Dodson, Ph.D., www.dodsonandross.com

Chris Donaghue, www.chrisdonaghue.com

Ducky Doolittle, www.duckydoolittle.com

Lauren Marie Fleming, www.laurenmariefleming.com

Charlie Glickman, Ph.D., www.charlieglickman.com and www.makesexeasy.com

Stella Harris, www.stellaharris.net

Tina Horn, www.whyarepeopleintothat.com

Shanna Katz, M.Ed., www.shannakatz.com

Ashley Manta, www.AshleyManta.com

Sunny Megatron, www.sunnymegatron.com

Mistress Simone, www.chicago-mistress.com

Allison Moon, www.talesofthepack.com

Dr. Emily Morse, www.sexwithemily.com

Emily Nagoski, Ph.D., www.thedirtynormal.com

JoEllen Notte, www.redheadbedhead.com

Jessica O'Reilly, Ph.D., www.sexwithdrjess.com

Gina Ogden, www.ginaogden.com

Sex Nerd Sandra, www.sexnerdsandra.com

Dawn Serra, www.dawnserra.com

Tristan Taormino, www.tristantaormino.com and www.puckerup.com

Jamye Waxman, www.jamyewaxman.com

Rebecca Jane Weinstein, www.rebeccajaneweinstein.com

Sex & Body Positive Coaches & Mental Health Professionals

The Open List

www.openingup.net/open-list

The Open List is a list of professionals (therapists, psychiatrists, psychologists, counselors, relationship and life coaches, doctors, lawyers, mediators, and alternative healthcare providers) who are experienced and knowledgeable about alternative sexuality and lifestyles, open relationships, polyamory, nonmonogamy, swinging, as well as BDSM, kink, leather, LGBTQIA communities, and other sexual minorities.

Kink Aware Professionals

www.ncsfreedom.org

The Kink Aware Professionals Directory (KAP) is a service offered by the National Coalition for Sexual Freedom (NCSF) dedicated to providing the community with a listing of psychotherapeutic, medical, legal, and other professionals who have stated that they are knowledgeable about and sensitive to diverse expressions of sexuality.

Acknowledgments

I couldn't ask for a better editor than Jess Haberman, whose good taste, smarts, and humor made writing my first book fun. My mentor and dear friend, Tristan Taormino, whose support and sage wisdom influence me every damn day. Lauren Marie Fleming and Tina Horn for recommending me to Quarto for this book. My best friends and adopted family, JoEllen Notte, Anne Hodder, Cyndi Darnell, Gene Reed, and Trey Ellett, who have supported me when they didn't have to, loved me when it wasn't easy, and cheered me on when I wanted to give up. Buck Angel who inspires me with every goddamn word that comes out of his mouth. Shannon Hardin and Jemma Rane, who encouraged me in the very beginning when no one else did. Paula Tiberius, who gave me my first writing job. My wonderful father, who, through it all, loved me and always had my back. Thank you to Justin for many, many things I can't list here. I'd like to acknowledge my fellow sex educators, whom I love and admire: Sandra Daugherty, Sunny Megatron, Ken Melvoin Berg, Charlie Glickman, Megan Andelloux, Jamye Waxman, Dr. Emily Morse, Ducky Doolittle, Ava Cadell, and Candida Royalle. I'd also like to thank the following people whose consistent support means so much: Tiffany Bowne, Dixie De La Tour, Ethan Feerst, Nathaniel V. Dust, Hudson Brooks, Marty Barrett, Sean Molloy, Laurie Kilpatrick, Nick Holmes, April Flores, Sheona McDonald, Sarah Tomchesson, Thor and Sandy Bruce, Dean Elliot, Denise Kraft and Melissa White. To those people who live in my heart: Phyllis Ostin, David Bowie, and Dina Bennett. And last but not least, my sweet little fur-baby, Hallerman Beyoncé Chase, who makes me smile every day.

About the Author

Sex educator, writer, and sex and intimacy coach Elle Chase is a graduate of the prestigious San Francisco Sex Information Sex Educator Training Program and a member of the American College of Sexologists. She is best known as the creator, curator, and editor of two award-winning and highly trafficked sexuality websites: www.ladycheeky.com (NSFW), and its companion editorial site www.smutforsmarties.com. Lady Cheeky was listed number one in *Cosmopolitan* and *Huffington Post*'s "Best Porn Sites for Women" lists, and was also named to Salon.com's "The Best of Tumblr Porn" list. Smut For Smarties has been *LA Weekly*'s choice as "Best Sex Blog" since 2013. Elle also serves as the director of education and lead sex educator at the Los Angeles Academy of Sex Education (www.laacademyofsex.com), where she offers master classes on sexuality, sexual health, and sexual lifestyles, taught by leading sex educators in their field and serving the community at large. Find Elle online at www.ellechase.com or on Twitter, Instagram, or Facebook @TheElleChase.

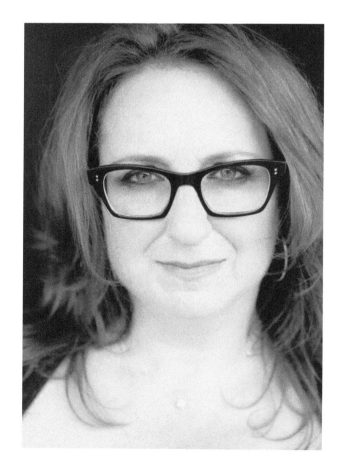

Index

Also Availables

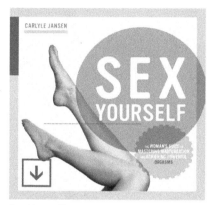

Sex Yourself
978-1-59233-679-1

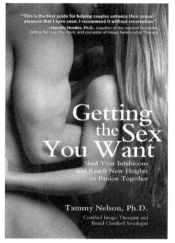

Getting the Sex You Want
978-1-59233-526-8

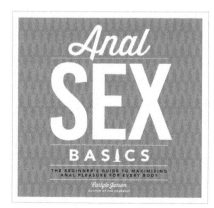

Anal Sex Basics
978-1-59233-703-3

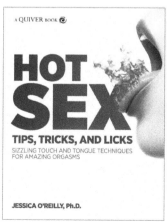

Hot Sex Tips, Tricks, and Licks
978-1-59233-535-0

CPSIA information can be obtained
at www.ICGtesting.com
Printed in the USA
JSHW051342070421
13295JS00010B/3

9 781592 337408